HOW TO ADD Sparkle & Pizzazz TO YOUR HEALTH PROMOTION PROGRAM

When work is your bliss, it is no longer work — Kathy Cash

When work is your bliss: it is no longer work.

Kathy Cash

HOW TO ADD

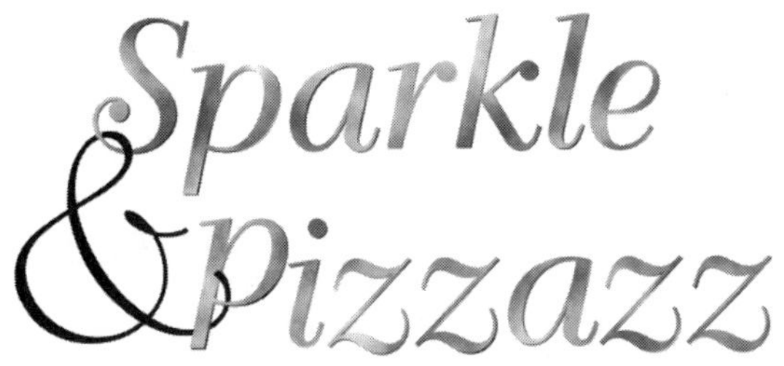

TO YOUR HEALTH PROMOTION PROGRAM

Kathy Cash, RN, CHPD

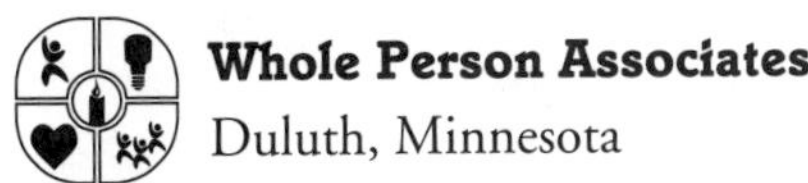

Whole Person Associates, Inc.
210 West Michigan
Duluth MN 55802-1908 218-727-0500
E-mail: books@wholeperson.com
Web site: http://www.wholeperson.com

How to Add Sparkle and Pizzazz to Your Health Promotion Program

Printed in the United States of America

10 9 8 7 6 5 4 3 2 1

Editorial Director: Susan Gustafson
Art Director: Joy Morgan Dey
Manuscript Editor: Kathy DeArmond
Production Manager: Paul Hapy

Library of Congress Cataloging-in-Publication Data

Cash, Kathy K.
How to add sparkle and pizzazz to your health promotion program : powerful programming tips to attract and motivate participants / Kathy K. Cash.
208 p. 27 cm.
Includes bibliographical references.
ISBN 1-57025-168-1 (pbk.)
1. Health promotion. I. Title.
RA427.8 .C38 1998
613—ddc21 98-8965
CIP

To my parents, who love me and worried.

To my husband, who loves me and pushed.

To my friends, who love me and were happy.

And to health promotion managers everywhere, for without you this book would not have been possible. A warmer, more giving group of people does not exist. This book is my attempt to distill what I have learned from you all over the years into what I hope is a useful tool to make your lives a little easier.

Table of contents

Fitness Programming

Nutrition Programming

Maternal/Child Programming

Programs and Activities for Healthy Aging

Resources

About the author

Kathy Cash is a registered nurse, a certified health promotion director, and a certified massage therapist with over eighteen years of health promotion experience. For fifteen of those years Kathy played an integral part in building the United States Air Force's health promotion program. After she retired as a lieutenant colonel, Kathy went on to design the first Department of Defense prevention program for a Fortune 500 health management organization. Kathy now lives in Edgewater, Florida, and provides professional speaking and consulting services on a wide variety of health promotion topics.

Kathy believes that over the years people lose touch with their bodies. They forget what it feels like to move freely and effortlessly. As a result, their entire interaction with the world around them is affected. Kathy provides customized services to help individuals and groups reach optimal physical and emotional performance through personalized counseling, massage services, and group seminars. Kathy also offers health promotion managers consultation on program design and problem solving. If you would like information about her workshops, seminars, and individualized consultations, please contact Kathy at:

Massage-U-Well
717 Charter Lane
Edgewater, FL 32141
Phone: 904-409-3398
Fax: 904-409-3326
E-mail: gcash@volusianet.net

Introduction

"Build It and They Will Come" does not apply to health education. It is common for great wellness programs to go unattended. This causes great frustration for novice and experienced managers alike. *How to Add Sparkle and Pizzazz to Your Health Promotion Program* focuses on administrative and programming strategies that create a structure and culture that supports each individual program and packs in participants.

Some of these strategies are so simple that they require only one or two paragraphs to explain. These suggestions appear in the "Quick Tips" chapter at the beginning of each section. Complex strategies receive more explanation in the subsequent chapters. I often include variations on the activities, as well as cross-references to activities and ideas in other chapters of the book. You can implement virtually all the ideas in this book on a modest working budget. To assist you in finding topics that best meet your needs, the chapters have been grouped into eight broad sections.

Raising Awareness, Changing Behavior, and Gaining Support
No health promotion program is effective without a strong support structure. Integral to this are creative marketing strategies, broad-based incentive programs, and strong management support. I assume in these chapters that health promotion managers know their target audiences and are willing to customize programs and services based on their diversity. But if you don't know your audience, don't worry! The next section includes strategies for learning about their needs.

Innovative Program Structure and Design
Decisions on what programs to offer (and how) should be strongly influenced by the customer. The customer is not just those attending the class, but also those who hired you (and why), who hold the purse strings, and who manage your customers. Customer-driven programs are actually easier to manage. If you truly listen to them, your customers will give you the programming answers you seek. Strategies for becoming customer-driven are included in this section, as well as specific tools to influence the learning process and effect long-term behavior change.

Health Fairs
What is your desired outcome? Health fair organizers don't ask this question often enough. As a result, health fairs become a "one size fits all" event—and consequently,

fit no one. This section defines nine types of health fairs. Health promotion managers select a target audience or specific community problem and then build a fair to address that need with the necessary depth to actually effect a desired health outcome or behavior change.

Fitness Programming
Fitness can be fun! This section has a wealth of ideas for turning mundane group fitness activities into high-energy social events that keep even the "couch potatoes" coming back for more. It is important that your programs not appeal just to the "jocks." Many of the activities play off our natural competitive natures but are structured to include people of all physical capabilities.

Nutrition Programming
It would be easy to eat well if we ate only at home and had no outside influences on our choices. This section provides strategies for encouraging healthy eating within the environment of today's average working person. It also gives easy-to-implement ideas for increasing awareness of healthy food selections and preparation.

Maternal/Child Programming
Many health habits learned at very early ages carry through well into adulthood. It's never too soon to begin instilling healthy ideas in children. Enjoyable and appealing programs and activities for preschoolers, elementary-age, preteens, and teenagers are described, as well as two excellent programs targeting new mothers' needs.

Programs and Activities for Healthy Aging
Issues of primary concern for today's aging populations are often not found in traditional health promotion programs. That is not to say that the traditional health promotion messages are not important. But integrating programs addressing the more personal needs of aging audiences will help capture this underserved population. This section provides programs and activities to address three often-overlooked areas: stages of life, encouraging independence and safety, and staying connected.

Resources
The resource section provides a compendium of organizations and companies that provide valuable resources and services for the "harried health promotion manager."

Raising Awareness, Changing Behavior, and Gaining Support

1 **Quick tips** 3

Sometimes you have a great program, but you need to get management and potential participants to pay attention. These quick tips give you techniques you can use with a wide variety of topics and approaches.

2 **Calendars** 10

Increase the likelihood recipients will actually keep and read your health promotion calendar of events by integrating target-audience-specific decorations, topics of interest, games, and incentives into a custom-designed template.

3 **Creative Program Linkages** 12

Our customers have a lot going on in their lives. When marketing a program, you must get their attention quickly. Create an immediate frame of reference to hook your target audience by linking programs with cultural interests, organizational mission, or national events.

4 **Wellness "Reality" Articles** 15

A series of real-life articles in an internal newsletter or a community newspaper constructs a "link" between wellness concepts and the lives of the target audience. Once involved in the "reality" articles, the reader seeks out supporting newsletter articles and learns about existing wellness services.

5 **Focus Groups** 18

Focus groups provide an opportunity to learn about your customers and their expectations for the health promotion program. Armed with that information, you can increase audience satisfaction and receive your customers' help in developing strategies for aligning services within the organizational, family, and social structures affecting them.

6 **Bogus Bucks** 26

Austere programming budgets make providing incentives to increase attendance and motivation difficult. "Bogus Bucks" is a creative strategy that expands limited resources while awarding a monetary value to a wide variety of wellness activities.

7 **Shift worker/Traveler/Multisite Incentives and Programming Strategies** 28

Reaching employees not available for on-site wellness programs requires creating significant target-audience motivation, as well as providing flexible self-study tools. The strategies outlined in this chapter can be developed totally in-house or blended with commercial products or community resources.

1 Quick Tips

Sometimes you have a great program, but you need to get management and potential participants to pay attention. These quick tips give you techniques you can use with a wide variety of topics and approaches.

Marketing

- **Seasonal entry blanks**

  Print health promotion program registration forms on colored paper in shapes appropriate to upcoming holidays: Christmas (ornaments, Santas); Halloween (jack-o-lanterns, ghosts, black cats); Independence Day (firecrackers, flags). Enter registrant information into a database; then use the registration forms as decorations in high traffic areas. The decorative entry blanks serve as a high-visibility reminder to others of the upcoming program.

  Variation: Make the registration forms in designs appropriate to the program topic: smoking cessation (cigarettes and cigars), nutrition (fruits and vegetables), substance abuse (wine bottles and syringes), fitness (running and bicycling figures).

- **Musical messages, groups, and competitions**

  Reinforce your wellness message with music. Play short taped music segments during anticipated quiet times. Make a humorous connection to the topic, such as "Smoke Gets in Your Eyes" during a tobacco-cessation program break; or actually design songs with a wellness message—for example, The lyrics of the old Motown hit "Stop in the Name of Love" could become "Stop (smoking, overeating, drinking, etc.) in the name of love before you break my heart." Look for local talent within your organization (or community). Offer them the opportunity to be your program's singing emissaries at special events or large gatherings.

  Variation: Have a competition or talent show for the best popular wellness songs or skits as part of a major event.

- **Wellness wiring diagram**

  When marketing within a corporate environment, especially to senior management, explain the major components of healthy living as if describing the departments of a large corporation. The chief executive officer supervises all of

Life Management. Senior presidents are in charge of the major components of health: Fitness, Emotional Health, and Relationships. Vice presidents or senior directors support topics, such as Nutrition, Exercise, Weight Management, Spiritual and Intellectual Growth, Interpersonal Relationships, Communication, and Parenting. Obviously, modify this strategy to reflect the structure of the organization being briefed, as well as the focus of your wellness programs. Many graphics software programs have wiring diagram capabilities (see the "wiring diagram" below).

WELLNESS WIRING DIAGRAM

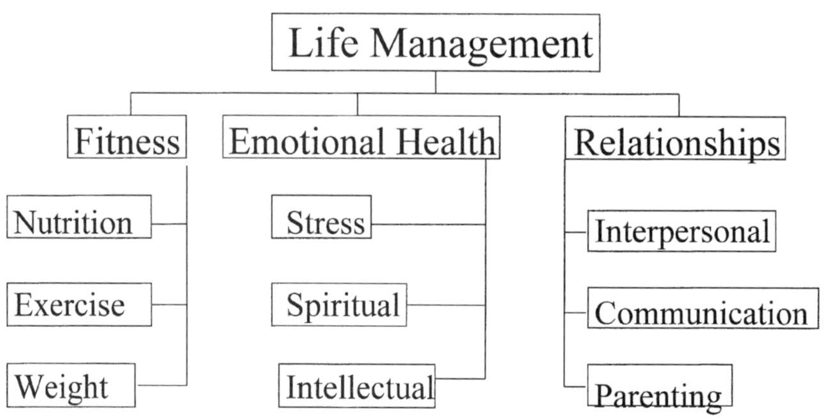

Variation: If you know the personalities involved in your briefing, try to inject a little humor. If Joe, a senior president, is a well-known runner, you could comment, "Obviously, the senior president of fitness must be Joe." Or use the opposite approach: If Mary is a well-known junk-food junkie, you might say, "I think it is safe to say that Mary is not the senior director for nutrition." Certainly, this approach should be used only if there is a congenial atmosphere and the briefer is fairly well known and accepted.

- **Corporate sponsorship**
  Expand program resources by seeking corporate sponsorship for specific programs and events. Many companies include community service as a corporate goal. They have committed funding or other resources to contribute to the well-being of the

community. Usually this service is confined to the geographic area near the organization itself; however, a number of large organizations feature ongoing wellness programs that they will take virtually anywhere upon request (see the Resources section).

On a smaller scale, local companies who seek the patronage of either your target audience or senior management may be eager to sponsor wellness events, especially if the events promise to be extensively marketed and attended. Sponsorship could be prizes, money, equipment, gift certificates, discounts, or volunteer workers. Start talking to local restaurants, department stores, grocery stores, movie theaters, sporting goods stores, car dealerships, and hospitals; but don't stop there. Seek out major suppliers or customers of your organization who are eager to cement working relationships.

Be sensitive that corporate sponsors have an agenda for supporting your event. Ask how they would like to be acknowledged for their support, and strive to help as long as it does not compromise your program's integrity or company policy. It should go without saying, but avoid soliciting sponsorship from alcohol or tobacco companies.

- **Target-audience writers/speakers**
  Look for people within your target audience who are willing to write or speak on the importance of the wellness program to them. These should be people still working towards a health goal: a young smoker who has tried to quit and relapsed, an overweight employee, a respected company retiree who survived a heart attack. The point of their article or speech is NOT to talk about theory or the how-tos of change. It should be about how they started down the road to where they are now, how hard it has been, perhaps what they have tried in the past that didn't work. Follow the article or speech with a promotion of an appropriate wellness program.

- **Creative graduation pictures**
  Graphically display the "cumulative" success of graduates from a behavior modification program. How many cigarette cartons will not be used in the next year by quitters in your tobacco-cessation class? Or what would a pile of fat look like to equal the total pounds lost by a weight management class? Or how far across a United States map would a line extend to equal the total miles run by a fitness group? Photograph the proud graduates with this display; and use it to market future programs in company newsletters, on bulletin boards, or as a slide in a briefing.

- **"Booby" prizes**
  There is no dishonor in losing, only in not trying. Make a point of acknowledging the efforts of all who participate in wellness competitions by rewarding the individual or team finishing last with a humorous prize. If possible, mirror the first place prize. For instance, turkeys are popular prizes around the holidays, so give a cornish game hen as a booby prize. If a dinner for two in a fancy restaurant is the first place prize, give a coupon for a free healthy selection TV dinner for last place.
- **"Wanted" posters**
  Promote your staff and program volunteers by imitating "Wanted" posters of the Old West. WANTED should be emblazoned in bold letters across the page above the traditional staff "mug shots". Below the picture in smaller letters, write the name of the individual(s), then the "crime." For instance, "Wanted—Jane Doe (fitness instructor) for Being Incredibly Fit. She was last seen running down Highway 50 in shorts and a T-shirt with the company logo. She is known to be recruiting new members for her gang. Call the Health Promotion Office at xxxx."

  It is sometimes easier to get a lot of volunteers who have only one specific responsibility versus a longtime commitment. Another version of the "wanted" poster is used to solicit volunteers. Summarize individual tasks in a series of short "classified ads" on the poster. For instance, "Wanted—volunteer to type up monthly calendar of events. Wanted—assistance with signing in participants at upcoming health fair. Wanted—aerobics leader for Thursday afternoon worksite fitness class, etc."
- **Positive program names**
  Maybe, to paraphrase Shakespeare, "A rose by any other name smells as sweet," but some program names have more impact than others. Do your program titles sound dry or academic? Try short, punchy titles with a descriptive subtitle. For instance, "Time to sign up for the next 'Kick Butt' Smoking Cessation Course, which starts on . . . " Avoid negative titles that imply attendees must have failed at something or they would not need the class. Try putting a positive spin on the titles. For example, instead of "Stress and Parenting" try "Parenting for the 90s" or "Parenting University."
- **Use of photographs and videos**
  Nothing says success better than pictures of happy participants. Photograph or videotape virtually everything about your program and use the best results in marketing presentations, especially to senior management. There is a side-benefit

for the health promotion manager: pictures showing the results of YOUR programming efforts are invaluable when looking for a job or proving your worth during negotiations for pay raises or budget increases. For similar reasons, maintain a file of all thank-yous and testimonials from delighted customers.

Incentives

- **Services**
  What types of home chores are common to your target audience? Is it housecleaning, getting the car washed, child care, lawn care? Lighten their load with service incentives. Program volunteers or the "losers" of a wellness competition relieve the "winner" of that chore for a specified period of time.
- **Special privileges**
  Find out what special privileges your target audience values. If someone in the organization controls the availability of that privilege, can it become a dedicated program incentive? A parking spot close to the office can be very popular, especially during the cold or rainy season. Casual days are increasingly popular. A special activity with the boss (breakfast or exercising) may appeal to some groups. Perhaps an employee can be relieved of an unpopular duty for a week or awarded special "King/Queen for a Day" treatment.
- **Registration fees/fund-raisers**
  Registration fees can be controversial. On the one hand they increase participants' commitment; on the other hand, they may turn some potential attendees away. As a rule, keep the registration fee nominal ($1–$5) and make its use as an incentive very obvious to participants. For instance, registration fees for a team competition could go toward T-shirts or small incremental incentives (if the program spans a number of weeks) or a certain amount could be split by the winning team as prize money.

  Fund-raisers come in many shapes: healthy-heart bake sales, car washes, raffles, services (see above), and more. Promote the fund-raiser as heavily as you would a wellness program. Make it fun for the volunteers as well as the participants. Encourage management to show their support by kicking off the fund-raiser.
- **Certificates**
  Develop a program identity that is maintained throughout the year. Reflect this theme in every initiative, piece of correspondence, briefing, item of promotional material, and the like. Develop a logo, program mascot, or motto. Have a "look"

to your material that is uniquely identified with the health promotion program. Design multipurpose certificates with the program logo. With today's computer programs, you can produce excellent certificates yourself; but even done commercially, it is surprisingly cheap. People love to display certificates, but to have meaning they cannot be used indiscriminately. Give the certificates out for achievements like graduating from special classes, volunteering, or reaching an important health goal. Where appropriate, make the presentation a special event. Certificates can be used for something as simple as a free apple or a healthy-heart cookbook included in a promotion for a nutrition class (which you would have given out anyway).

Ways to involve management

- **Supervisors as relief for employees**
  Employees always prefer to participate in wellness programs during the workday; but in many work environments this is extremely difficult. When employees must attend programs during off-duty time, demonstrate the value management places on wellness programs. Occasionally have supervisors stand in for employees at the worksite in order for them to attend special worktime programs. This supervisor coverage could be conducted as a special privilege, through a raffle, or on a rotational basis.

- **Supervisor award program**
  Encourage supervisors to foster a healthy workplace by creating an ongoing award program recognizing their efforts. Criteria for judging the most deserving supervisor could include encouraging personnel participation in wellness programs, establishing a worksite healthy-snack bar, providing flextime for exercising, purchasing ergonomic office equipment, having the greatest percentage of employees enrolled in company 401K programs, or achieving the best safety record.

  Variation: Expand this idea to include all employees who have contributed ideas to improve organizational health. Consider channeling their efforts towards an identified problem such as worksite safety, ergonomic issues, or environmental stressors.

- **Travel files**
  If senior leaders are required to travel frequently, find out from their secretaries if they routinely carry a "travel" file. Travel files are usually a variety of work-related documents used by executives as reading material during trips. Determine

the process for providing input to this file. "Feed" it with quick-read wellness articles and information. Include industry statistics on the value of health promotion programs. Remember, these are busy people. Do not overwhelm them with too much information! In fact, for complex topics, provide a summary page highlighting the key points of the article.

- **Senior management video**

  Messages from management supporting wellness have an obvious advantage in program marketing. Videos make it possible to replay the message without infringing on the busy time of the senior leader. While the basic goal of the film is to illustrate the leaders' support, try to lead into the dialogue with one or more senior leaders shown participating in a wellness activity (taking a brisk walk, playing tennis, eating a healthy meal, etc.). Then one or more of the leaders share their personal wellness journey. Maybe they were workaholics and eventually realized they needed to spend more time with their families or exercising.

  Variations: As part of this video, or as a second video, show the formal or informal leaders of the blue-collar workforce sharing similar feelings. Tape an organizational fitness video with managers as the background exercisers.

2 Calendars

Increase the likelihood recipients will actually keep and read your health promotion calendar of events by integrating target-audience-specific decorations, topics of interest, games, and incentives into a custom-designed template.

Many health and wellness customers are actually interested in programs, but miss the program advertisements altogether; hear about them too late; or hear about them, then forget. Calendars of events sent to individual members or small segments of the target audience are helpful only if they are read and retained for reference. A calendar of events should be considered a promotional piece and designed with just as much care and imagination as any marketing brochure.

Goals

To increase readership and retention of health promotion program calendar of events

To raise awareness of and participation in health promotion programs

Target audience

All types

Process

- Identify specific target audiences who will receive the calendar.
- Design a standardized calendar template that, in addition to essential information on all monthly events, allows room for decoration and other types of information in margins and unused areas of the template.
- Identify individuals knowledgeable about the likes and dislikes of the various target audiences in areas such as these:

  entertainment

  artwork

  cooking preferences

  hobbies

  special interests

- Each month, provide a high-quality copy of the calendars to the volunteers to customize for their assigned target audience. If the calendar is computer-generated, provide a copy on disk for customizing. Customization can also be done by freehand drawing, typing, or "cut and paste" decoration.
- Volunteers return the customized calendars to the health promotion office by a predetermined suspense date for reproduction and distribution.
- Ideas for customization:

  coupons

    food items

    popular restaurants

    an incentive to be claimed at an upcoming health promotion event

  short promotional statement about specific events that have a special relevancy to the target audience

  schedules of popular events: sporting events, concerts, club meetings

  sales at frequented business establishments

  healthy-heart recipes: ethnic, for children, snacks for singles

  borders or decorations specific to the audience
- Other ideas for increasing readership and retention:

  "Find the ___" contest—a simple strategy where recipients search for a small object hidden somewhere on the calendar. The object can be anything: an apple, health promotion program logo, etc. The first person to find the object and notify the health promotion office wins, or a small incentive is given to anyone who finds the object.

  In a worksite program, try placing a different employee identification number somewhere on the calendar each month. The number should be small but readable, and not in the same spot each month. If the employee(s) comes forward by a certain date he or she gets some sort of incentive.

  Puzzles are popular with many people. Develop your own or buy a book or software program with ready-made puzzles. Incorporate a wellness theme or information found in the contents of the calendar. Offer an incentive for correctly filled out puzzles.

Cross-Reference: Chapter 6, Bogus Bucks; Chapter 8, Quick Tips (Wellness Crossword Puzzle)

3 Creative Program Linkages

Our customers have a lot going on in their lives. When marketing a program, you must get their attention quickly. Create an immediate frame of reference to hook your target audience by linking programs with cultural interests, organizational mission, or national events.

Today's customers expect Madison Avenue marketing tactics which quickly establish product relevancy, often with strong humorous overtones. Health educators need not change program content to get an audience in the door. Instead, constantly strive to update marketing strategies with unique and timely messages.

Goals

To provide creative strategies for marketing traditional health promotion programs

To increase interest and appeal of health promotion programs

Target audience

All types

Process

- This process should be a component of the overall structure for scheduling health promotion activities.
- Create a timeline (preferably reflecting an entire year) of planned health promotion activities by

  blocking off on the timeline programs that must be offered on a specific date;

  noting programs that must be held within a specific time frame but have flexibility on the date; and

  reflecting programs that can be offered at any time.
- Compare the program timeline to the following:

  special recognitions

    national health observances

    national holidays

cultural holidays or recognitions

seasons

events in the news

popular entertainment icons or events

unique events or areas of interest within an organization or group

- Look for ways to link the program to one or more of these events.

  Are there ethnic or cultural observances that can be linked to programs targeting that group?

  "Black Heritage Month"—African American health fair

  Cinco de Mayo—healthy-heart Mexican cooking

  Some obvious links can be made to national holidays, but also look for creative links by analyzing the meanings behind a holiday or the characteristics of the individual being honored. Free-flow brainstorming with a small group of people is very effective here.

  Valentines Day—heart health, improving personal relationships

  Fourth of July—"independence" from smoking

  Washington's Birthday—"Don't tell a lie . . . truth in labeling." February is Dental Health Month as well: "The father of our country could have avoided this [picture of wooden teeth] if he had practiced better dental hygiene."

  Lincoln's Birthday—"Everyone experiences depression, even President Lincoln" as a lead-in for an emotional health program.

  Halloween—costumed fun run

- Look for links that can be used in promoting the overall health promotion program.

  Columbus Day—Discover your health promotion office.

  New Year's Day—Made any resolutions to improve your health in the New Year? We can help.

- Use your brainstorming group to create programming or marketing ideas linked to the seasons and special interest areas of the target audience.

  Summer—heat injuries, allergies, swimming safety

  Olympics—fitness, wellness competition

Academy awards—Be a star in your family: quit smoking.

Miss America competition—skin care, beauty starts from within

- Make a connection to a popular movie playing in the theaters.
- Juxtapose two dissimilar but recognizable items/persons:

  Lincoln and depression

  razor and a heart (human concern/personal torment)

  deer crossing sign with red nose on deer to promote holiday safety

- Incorporate the responsibilities of a department into a marketing theme. I once saw a helicopter maintenance shop promote Dental Health Month with this theme: "Choppers [picture of helicopter blades attached to flying sets of teeth] will play a big part in Dental Health Week."
- Even after your marketing strategies have been mapped out for the year, be flexible enough to take advantage of an unexpected event that has caught the attention of your audience. Examples:

  An employee's heart attack can be incorporated into the existing plan. When a heart-attack survivor returns to work, invite him or her to talk about unhealthy behaviors that may have contributed to the attack, as a prelude to a coronary-artery risk-reduction program. Ask the employee to promote a heart-health program in advance to encourage attendance.

  Regardless of his guilt or innocence, it's a fact that awareness and interest in spouse-abuse programs was markedly raised during the O. J. Simpson murder trial.

4 Wellness "Reality" Articles

A series of real-life articles in an internal newsletter or a community newspaper constructs a "link" between wellness concepts and the lives of the target audience. Once involved in the "reality" articles, the reader seeks out supporting newsletter articles and learns about existing wellness services.

Often, newsletter articles tend toward generalization and theory rather than practical application. Wellness information must make a connection with the target audience's personal lives; otherwise, they fail to appreciate its importance to them.

Goals

To market wellness services

To illustrate wellness concepts meaningful to the target audience

To demonstrate that lifestyle changes are attainable

Target audience

All types

Process

- Obtain two volunteers from the target audience who are representative of its major subgroups. Example: If the target audience comprises both males and females, both blue-collar and white-collar employees, with dominant age groups 20s and 30s, and ethnic groups white and African American, a good choice for two volunteers would be a white male blue-collar employee in his early 20s and an African-American female white-collar employee in her late 30s.
- Conduct the full battery of wellness assessments available to the reading audience, including the following:

  health risk appraisal and needs assessment

  fitness tests

  health screenings

  counselings

- Meet with each volunteer individually to
  - discuss findings;
  - determine personal health goals;
  - review available health promotion services and strategies to support goals;
  - enroll in appropriate programs; and
  - define parameters of information that volunteers are comfortable sharing with the public.
- Commit with volunteers to meet at set intervals to
  - monitor progress toward health goals;
  - counsel as needed to assist volunteers towards these goals; and
  - review information for upcoming articles.
- Plan a calendar of articles chronicling the volunteers' progress, setbacks, obstacles to success, and strategies to overcome any problems encountered as they progress through the programs.
- The frequency of articles should be at least once a month, to keep up general interest; the entire series should run between six months and a year.
- The initial article should
  - provide sufficient personal and professional information on each volunteer to elicit a sense of connection from the reading audience;
  - include lifestyle issues, especially if they are commonly found in the target audience;
  - explain the evaluations conducted on the volunteers and the appropriate findings;
  - emphasize that these same services are available to reading audiences;
  - outline the agreed-upon goals and general strategies; and
  - explain the frequency and type of articles to expect in the future relating back to the progress of the volunteers.
- Subsequent articles should include a brief summary of volunteers' overall progress, but should focus on only one or two health topics per article.
- Attempt to achieve a "soap opera" tone to the articles:
  - Discuss life events in the context of how they (positively or negatively) affect the volunteers' progress.

What is going to happen next? Will they overcome problems slowing their progress? How did they celebrate a milestone?

Finish with a "teaser" paragraph about the topic of the next article.

- Tie other information articles in each edition of the newsletter to issues relating to volunteers. Example: If a volunteer is trying to quit smoking and has a relapse, a general discussion about how smoking triggers played a part in his or her setback would be appropriate in the main article. Include a second article on smoking triggers—how to identify them and develop strategies to overcome them. A line in the main volunteer article directs the reader to the accompanying article: "For more information on how to identify triggers, see the article entitled '___' on the next page of this newsletter."
- The final article of the series should compare the volunteers' lifestyle and health status at the beginning of the program to their current status.
- Even if they have not achieved their goals, the article should emphasize what progress they've made, what they have learned, and how they are committed to follow through. This is important! We learn from our failures; but many people are afraid to start a lifestyle modification program out of fear of failure.

  Attempt to estimate health years gained as a result of the lifestyle changes; but don't ignore the more intangible benefits, such as improved self-esteem and increased energy.

  When a volunteer fails to reach one or even most of his or her goals, put a positive spin on this. Thomas Edison, who failed in more than one thousand experiments to invent the light bulb, was asked how it felt to fail so many times. Edison snapped, "I didn't fail one thousand times. I discovered one thousand ways that wouldn't work."

  Note: There is a frequent side-benefit for the volunteers. As a result of their notoriety in the "reality" articles, they will soon have a tremendous support system of people who are encouraging them toward their goals on a daily basis.

Cross-Reference: Chapter 14, Needs Assessment

5 Focus Groups

Focus groups provide an opportunity to learn about your customers and their expectations for the health promotion program. Armed with that information, you can increase audience satisfaction and receive your customers' help in developing strategies for aligning services within the organizational, family, and social structures affecting them.

To assume that a target audience needs a certain type of health promotion program is at least presumptuous, and that assumption ultimately leads to failure of your program if the target audience does not value your choice. Individuals interpret and react to information based on influences going back to childhood and evolving with changing life experiences at home, at work, and among their peers. Health promotion managers must be willing to shake off preconceived notions of what their program must be, climb inside their audiences' reality, and design programs from that perspective.

Goals

To gain insights into the cultural and life experiences of a specific target audience

To design health promotion products and services that best meet customer expectations and needs

Target audience

All types

Process

- Most health promotion programs include some form of health-risk appraisal to evaluate individual health risks. Even when the appraisal compiles a group composite, it rarely provides insights as to what causes individual self-destructive behaviors and how people want the health promotion program to help them change. Group needs assessments accomplish that goal, and focus groups are an invaluable resource in an overall needs-assessment strategy.
- Health promotion focus groups typically include five to eight people who

represent an audience sharing certain demographics such as ethnicity, culture, religion, gender, age, work, or economic status.

- The purpose of a health promotion focus group is to gain insights about common influences on a group that affect their decisions about health and their perceptions of the health promotion program. The information gathered makes it possible to anticipate how a target audience will react to wellness initiatives.

  As representatives of a larger target audience, focus-group members can stimulate excitement about the entire health and wellness program and be instrumental in reducing resistance to program or organizational changes. Focus-group involvement in program planning and the implementation process encourages target audience acceptance.

  The fresh ideas and perspectives gathered in a focus group provide program planners with new marketing ideas and alternatives to meeting wellness goals.

- Prior to focus-group meetings,

  Set focus group goals, which could include:

    developing program and marketing strategies;

    learning audience perceptions of health promotion, healthy living, and its benefit;

    determining health promotion products and services needed by the audience;

    learning how the audience uses products and services currently provided;

    determining which current health promotion products and services do not meet needs;

    gaining insights as to how current services, products, and the like could be modified to better meet needs;

    gathering specific recommendations to improve product or service quality.

  Plan how to gather the desired information. Are there informal leaders, individuals who are most at risk, or people who offer your target audience support and friendship who could represent this group's interests?

  Identify any inviolate program areas that are not open for discussion.

- All focus groups need a facilitator to:

  Help group members reach their goals through

    recommending strategies and problem-solving techniques

researching questions posed by the group

helping the group get around obstacles or impasses

Attend the meetings but function as neither leader nor member (although he or she may occasionally participate in discussions)

Maintain neutrality to ensure issues receive an impartial review

Encourage open discussion through well-placed nonjudgmental observations

Help control difficult people or situations that may arise

Ensure that all members participate and that no one person dominates discussions

Act as liaison to health promotion staff and other key individuals to present information and assist in drawing conclusions

Act as timekeeper, but let the group decide if discussion should go longer or postpone

- It typically takes a focus group between one and three sessions to gather all the information needed.
- If the group does not object, it is a good idea to tape sessions; ideas will be coming fast and furious.
- Activities for the first meeting should include

  explaining the purpose of the team, the goals of the health promotion program, the desired outcome of their efforts, and the use to be made of the information;

  establishing a solid working relationship among members. Many of the ice-breaker activities found in Whole Person Associates' structured exercise manuals have excellent ideas for warm-up activities;

  sharing strengths and weaknesses brought to the group;

  seeking to establish ground rules for compliments/disagreements.
- General rules:

  Use an agenda, including topics with definitions and reasons for their discussion, presenters, estimated time for each item, and scheduled breaks.

  Keep a record of all discussions.
- Strongly discourage people from being called away from the meeting (phone messages, etc.).
- Use a flip chart to keep information from getting lost or forgotten, to allow

everyone to see the same information, to let people know their ideas have been heard, and to allow the group to review its work from earlier in the session or earlier sessions.

- Brainstorming is an excellent tool to stimulate a free flow of ideas. Ask an open-ended question geared toward providing insight into some component of the group's goals.
- When a question is posed to the group and they come to an agreement on an answer, explore the causal factors that make it true. What are the biases, beliefs, obstacles, and such that cause their answer to be true.

  How strong are the various influences of these causes on the problem?

  Do you need any additional information not available to the group to verify the influence of these causes?

  Are there obvious changes that would eliminate causes? What steps can you take to eliminate less obvious causes?
- Once the root causes for a behavior have been identified, the focus group can help develop an appropriate solution(s) to resolve the problem.

  Clearly define the problem, the need it creates, or the opportunity it affords the health promotion program.

  Decide the goals (desired outcomes) of your solution. Set criteria to help evaluate potential solutions.

  Identify constraints, such as money, technical limits, and management issues.

  Generate alternatives. What are minor solutions that could be tried immediately versus more complex solutions that may require time?

  Evaluate the alternatives against the group's defined criteria for a solution and narrow them down to two or three options.

  Discuss possible disadvantages, negative consequences, and opportunities for misunderstanding.

  Select the best overall solution.

  Establish a follow-up plan to evaluate the progress and success of the proposed solution.
- As you gain insights into the customers' expectations, be sure you can state their expectations completely and concisely.

- Once the changes are made, the challenge then becomes how to package and/or market these changes to excite these group representatives and their leaders about the new and improved health promotion program. Ask them these questions:

  Do they need to see the idea in action?

  Do they need to see data that is relevant to them?

  Do they need to talk to people involved in the change?

  Make accommodations to their concerns as necessary.

  Be able to respond with data if asked questions. Do your homework on the topic.

- Quick techniques to deal with group problems.

  When trying to find a way around tangents, directionless discussions, or resistance to progress, try the following statements:

  "Let's review our purpose for this group and make sure it's clear."

  "What do we need to do to move on?"

  "What is holding us up?"

  "Are we stuck because we missed or left something incomplete?"

  "Everyone write down what we think is needed to move on to the next stage."

  With overbearing or dominating participants, it is important to reinforce agreement that no area is sacred. Get the team to agree that "balance of participation" is important. Get the problem participant(s) to agree up front that members must understand everything about an issue. Ask for cooperation and understanding privately as needed. Impose a structure on discussion of key issues. Be a gatekeeper: "We've heard from you, _____. Let's hear what others have to say."

  Structure discussions to encourage reluctant or shy people to participate. Ask for written-out responses. When possible, give the individual a task or assignment. As gatekeeper, look directly at the individual when asking for further comment.

  When dealing with an individual who demands unquestioned acceptance of an opinion as fact, try these approaches:

  Ask, "Is what you said opinion or a fact? Do you have data?"

  State, "Let's accept what you say as 'possible,' but let's also get some data to test it."

  Have group agree on the importance of making data-driven recommendations.

Encourage active listening skills early on. When no one acknowledges an individual's statement, support the discounted person:

"It sounds like that is important to you and we aren't giving it enough consideration."

Talk off-line to individuals who frequently discount others.

Digressions and tangents may be innocent or due to a desire to avoid a sensitive topic. Use a written agenda with time limits on each topic. Direct conversation back on track:

"We've strayed from the topic, which was _____."

"We've had trouble sticking to this point. Is there something about it that makes it so easy to avoid?"

Feuding team members usually have a history of issues with each other prior to the focus group. Require an up-front agreement between combatants on behavior in the meetings. When confrontations occur during a meeting, get adversaries to discuss off-line . . . offer to facilitate. Push them to a contract about their behavior.

- Other tips for stimulating discussion.

Direct an open-ended question to a specific person to obtain his or her input.

Offer a general question to the whole group so that anyone can volunteer a response.

Returning a question back to the person who asked it is especially effective when the person asking the question appears to have more to say than the question indicates:

"John, you asked how to ______. Where would you start?"

Deflecting a question to another person is an excellent technique for bringing in noncontributors or for giving a person with data a chance to respond directly to the question:

"Jane, you've been working in that area for awhile; how would you respond to Jim's question?"

Recognize constructive participation—people repeat what has been reinforced:

give verbal feedback—"Good," "That's right," "Thank you, that was very enlightening," "Excellent point," etc.;

make an approving expression or gesture;

encourage expression of incomplete or roughly formulated thoughts/ideas; allow proposals or ideas to be fully developed before moving on.

- A focus group should always be aware of their decision-making options.

  Poll their opinions on a topic of discussion.

  Test for consensus. Does everyone seem to agree? Is anyone unsure?

  Can the decisions or recommendations be validated by data?

  Watch for these:

  minority decisions not empowered by larger group

  too frequent recourse to "majority rules"

  a lack of discussion being considered approval

- After each focus group meeting, analyze the results:

  What improvements did customers suggest?

  What were the trends in customer problems?

  Look for commonalties.

  Did you see any problems not identified by the customers?

  With whom can you check the validity of your conclusions (other customers, leaders, informed participants)?

- Use the information you gain from these focus groups to:

  develop key leaders' awareness of problem;

  define the desired change carefully;

  break down the proposed solution into implementation steps;

  assign implementation responsibilities and decide who needs to be consulted;

  get word out before rumors start . . . validate solution with target audience;

  determine realistic timelines;

  ask yourself:

  How will you track status towards completion?

  How will you monitor impact?

  How will you deal with unexpected problems?

Have you done everything to optimize success?

Can the lessons learned about the change be used elsewhere?

Cross-Reference: Chapter 12, Programming Decision Matrix; Chapter 14, Needs Assessment

6 Bogus Bucks

Austere programming budgets make providing incentives to increase attendance and motivation difficult. "Bogus Bucks" is a creative strategy that expands limited resources while awarding a monetary value to a wide variety of wellness activities.

Not surprisingly, money consistently ranks at the top as the most valued incentive. Play money is an excellent alternative to stretch a tight budget while putting a higher perceived value on traditional products and services used in incentive programs.

Goals

To optimize resources dedicated to program incentives

To encourage and reinforce behavior change

To increase program participation

Target audience

All types

Process

- Design the "bogus bucks" so they can be economically produced but not easily forged. A few examples:

  number the dollars sequentially

  use a special paper with a specific thickness, color, watermark

  use a unique color of ink

  require a signature or stamp for the "bucks" to be cashed
- Identify all incentive program products and services available to customers. Some possibilities:

  T-shirts, mugs, sports bottles, refrigerator magnets, etc.

  housecleaning, car wash, lawn care, taking over an office responsibility, etc.

  discounts at local restaurants, movie theater passes, grocery store coupons, etc.
- Place a "bogus bucks" value on each product, service, or privilege. A good rule

of thumb is $10 worth of bogus bucks for every $1 worth of value:

a $2 coffee mug would be worth $20 in bogus bucks;

a house cleaning with an estimated value of $40 would be worth $400 in bogus bucks;

a special parking place for a month, estimated value of $40, would be worth $400 in bogus bucks.

- Develop a list of alternatives for earning health promotion bogus bucks and place a value on each:

  attending a program

  winning or placing in a fitness, or some other type of wellness competition

  achieving an established health goal

  accomplishing voluntary screenings or assessments

  practicing healthy behaviors observed by a designated oversight official

  Consider "weighting" programs that target corporate goals with more points.
- Display all incentives with their bogus buck price tags.
- Include the bogus buck value of all programs and activities as part of the marketing campaign.

Variations

Establish a special value for attending wellness programs offered prior to Christmas/ Hanukkah holiday season.

Help reduce holiday stress by providing a gift-wrapping service to busy employees for a preestablished number of accrued bogus bucks.

Establish gift-wrapping stations in lunchroom or during office Christmas party.

Cross-Reference: Chapter 1, Quick Tips (Incentives)

7 Shift Worker/Traveler/Multisite Incentives and Programming Strategies

Reaching employees not available for on-site wellness programs requires creating significant target-audience motivation, as well as providing flexible self-study tools. The strategies outlined in this chapter can be developed totally in-house or blended with commercial products or community resources.

Shift workers and geographically separated employees are rarely provided easy access to health promotion programs; yet by virtue of their isolation, they tend to have some of the most significant lifestyle problems and health risks.

Goals

To improve the access of geographically separated audiences and shift workers to wellness program information

To motivate geographically separated audiences and shift workers to avail themselves of health promotion products and services

Target audience

Employees not available for traditional daytime on-site health promotion programs

Process

- Recording in-house programs is one obvious answer to reaching underserved audiences; but health promotion staff are often intimidated by the prospect, fearing they will produce a substandard product. Although the more professional the equipment the better the product, some of these strategies can work with amateur audio- or videotaping equipment. If voices are understandable, and in the case of a camcorder, visual aids are legible, employees receiving these tapes appreciate the effort and are surprisingly forgiving. Obviously, commercially made audiocassettes and videos are an option. Some of these strategies require at least an internal computer network within the company.
- Make it possible

  for employees who are on the road for significant periods of time to play audiotape programs in the car while traveling between assignments and audio- and videotapes in a hotel room or at home;

and for shift workers and those at other sites to play the tapes at home or at work.

Make it convenient by

having audiocassette and videotape players that employees can sign out for a day or a week;

setting up audiocassette and videotape players in quiet corners of the lunchroom or nearby spots;

providing a list to traveling employees of the many hotels that make available televisions with videotape players.

- It is easy to put off playing such tapes. An incentive program is very valuable to encourage listening/watching the programs:

  to validate the tape has been played, develop a basic quiz on the information;

  include the quiz with each tape when it is mailed or checked out;

  to receive the incentive, the employee fills out the quiz and sends it in to the health promotion office.

- For multisite organizations, peer education is not only popular, it is also highly effective because the instructor understands and can relate to the audience.

  Select programs that can be taught by lay instructors through a commercial "train-the-trainer" program or by the health promotion staff. The best choices for such programs are usually nontechnical, are very focused, and deal with one issue. A few examples of such programs are: smoking cessation, healthy-heart cooking, time management, running.

  Support groups run by the participants offer a practical forum for members to share useful information and help each other problem-solve obstacles to achieving program goals. While it is not necessary for a knowledgeable professional to be in attendance at every meeting, periodic attendance or long-distance consultation via telephone will help ensure members stay focused and are productive.

  In either case, the peer groups should be supported by the health promotion office with appropriate commercial or locally developed videos and/or manuals.

- Video conferencing is rapidly becoming recognized as an economical way to bring many people together without the expense of traveling to one site.

Many multisite companies have video conferencing capabilities or are considering it. Where it is being considered, help with the justification. Do your homework. Show the economic benefits to be derived from getting health promotion information in front of more of their employees. Commit to dedicating a portion of your budget to help defray operating costs.

Local universities and hospitals frequently have videoconferencing capabilities. If any of your sites are near their network, approach these institutions and ask to rent time (if they do not offer it for free). It may not be possible to reach every site through their network, but you might be able to reach some. Those sites not near a video site can listen to the audio portion of the program via telephone hookup.

- Computer networks offer a wealth of opportunities for health promotion staff to reach out anywhere in the world and touch their customers. While most health promotion personnel are relatively inexperienced in computer networks and the Internet, if your company has a network there are very likely personnel on staff in the computer department who can advise and assist you towards accomplishing your goals.

  Virtually all companies with computer networks have some method to electronically mail messages to individuals or select groups. Use this forum for sending out a wellness newsletter or general promotion messages on upcoming programs. If you maintain a database of employees with specific wellness interest areas, you can target this group with the appropriate information.

  Many internal computer networks have a bulletin board capability. Bulletin boards can also be a source for posting upcoming events. Bulletin boards can be set up as a question-answer forum. Such forums can be made anonymous if that is a need. If you can get network rights to health promotion learning programs and self-assessments, they can be posted on the computer network bulletin board and accessed at any company terminal.

  Many commercial companies and some United Way agencies have health promotion information adapted to the computer. It is necessary to determine how reproduction rights for these products are granted for use on computer networks. If the target audience is large enough, consider funding a health educator consultant to develop your company's own line of health education information to put on the network (and reproduce in hard copy). In the long run, this strategy could save money since the cost of buying the rights to commercial information pieces would be eliminated. Also, well-written internally developed information pieces add to the appearance of professionalism of the overall program.

The Internet has become an invaluable repository of health promotion information, but many companies have legitimate concerns about allowing employees access to the Internet at work. Explore the Internet on your own and seek out the sites that best meet your program needs. Depending on the source, some of these sites may allow you to reproduce their entire site onto your company's internal network for free or at a nominal charge. Management should not object to this arrangement.

Another strategy is to compile the Internet addresses of the good health and wellness sites and make them available to employees. Encourage employees to visit these sites on their own time by developing simple quizzes that ask questions about information found at the Internet sites. Offer an incentive or reward for visiting the sites and successfully filling out the respective quizzes.

- Most community hospitals offer health and wellness programs as a community service. These programs are not intended to be a source of revenue. Any registration fees are usually nominal and only help defray costs.

  Approach one or two local community hospitals near your target audience and offer some (or all) of the organizational funds earmarked for your remote sites' health promotion program. The money could be paid in one lump sum each year, or in increments each quarter. In return, the hospital opens up all (or select) health promotion programs to your audience for free. The hospital provides their calendar of events for dissemination.

  Just offering the hospital a set amount of money is usually preferable to being billed for each individual attending a program. Billing creates an administrative burden the hospitals' staff probably can't handle. It would be appropriate to request copies of program registration sheets to track patterns of program use. The amount of money given in the next period could be adjusted if significantly more or fewer people attend than anticipated.

- Stretch your budget. Look around for other companies who offer wellness programs (or would like to) located near your remote site(s). Approach them with an offer to share resources. Perhaps they can sponsor one program in a quarter and your organization can sponsor a second on a different topic.

  Whether both companies' employees attend the same program or it is offered twice at two locations, there is still a considerable cost savings. Other than the cost of handouts, the administrative costs and expense of bringing in a speaker are of much more financial significance than the number of attendees.

- Overseas branches of multisite organizations present a unique challenge to a stateside health promotion staff. Some of the above suggestions may help, but here are a few more ideas to explore.

  Overseas Army, Navy, and Air Force military installations with a medical treatment facility usually employ at least one health promotion manager and have access to other trained medical professionals. The health promotion staff may be able to open the doors to their existing programs to your organization. Even if there are restrictions on that alternative, members of the medical staff may be eager to teach on their off-duty time for a consulting fee. Often military personnel have spouses who are medical professionals but who are not working during the overseas tour. Many of these people would be excited at the opportunity to earn some extra money teaching and providing other wellness services.

  Health promotion is not unique to the United States. There are health and wellness associations in many other countries, just as there are here. Hospitals or universities near your sites may be a resource. A good place to start looking for help is the International Institute of Health Promotion (see the Resources section).

  If you find no health promotion resources near your overseas branches, but do have someone on-site who can provide logistical support, consider forming a health promotion and education association. It may not be as difficult as it sounds if there are employee spouses there with some medical expertise and/or a local hospital. Continuing education for nurses and other nonphysician professionals is not as prevalent as it is in the United States. There may be surprising interest in bringing together like-minded professionals to share cultural information and pool resources to offer health and wellness programs for the American community as well as the local nationals.

Cross-Reference: Chapter 6, Bogus Bucks; Chapter 11, Phone Clinics; Chapter 15, Databases; Section 8, Resources (International Institute of Health Promotion)

Innovative Program Structure and Design

16 **Health Promotion Committees** **63**
A successful health promotion program requires top to bottom involvement of major target audiences and seeks out potential programming partners. Learn how to effectively structure and manage health promotion committees and how to use subcommittees to enhance efficiency and encourage involvement of key players.

8 Quick Tips

These quick tips offer ideas for games, information dissemination, and creative visual aids to enhance the learning process and make old programs seem lively and new.

- **Wellness crossword puzzle**

At the beginning of a wellness program, offer attendees a unique note-taking tool: a crossword puzzle whose answers will be given out during the presentation. Puzzle clues highlight the most important points of the presentation. Encourage even closer attention by rewarding attendees who successfully fill out the puzzle at the end of the program. A variation to this idea can be used with wellness newsletters. Puzzle answers are found within the content of the newsletter. There are many easy-to-operate computer software programs available for designing crossword puzzles.

- **Wellness Jeopardy**

Wellness Jeopardy works equally well as a competition within an organization or a school. Designed along the lines of the popular television show, categories can be broad, such as the components of health (tobacco, stress, nutrition, fitness, etc.), or topics targeting a certain audience. For instance, a kids' competition could be "Drug Jeopardy" with such categories as tobacco, alcohol, inhalants, street drugs, and weight loss drugs. Other focused topics could be workplace priorities or desired behaviors (communication, benefit plans, safety, ergonomics, etc.). Ideas for questions can come from focus groups, the Internet, library, past programs, or company statistics department.

- **Health promotion debates**

This strategy is especially effective in a multisession behavior modification program. After the facilitator has discussed the positive benefits of changing the undesirable behavior and the class has begun practicing the various strategies for changing a behavior, invariably there comes a point where some of the attendees are feeling anxiety, hostility, or concerns about their ability to effect long-term change. Divide the class into those who want to defend the old behavior and those who want to convince the others to change. If the group is not equally divided, ask someone to take the opposing view and defend it to the best of his or her ability. As long as the debate addresses issues effecting changing behavior, allow the class to go in whatever direction with the discussion they desire. The facilitator acts as moderator and stimulates discussion or refocuses the group as necessary. This is also an effective strategy for discussing controversial organizational issues or resistance to change.

- **Bulletin boards**

Put organizational wellness bulletin boards in high-traffic areas. Develop an accordion file with health and wellness articles, program promotions, cartoons, healthy-heart recipes, wellness brochures, and pictures of past wellness events. Organize the file by dedicating each pocket to a different wellness category, for example, fitness, nutrition, stress. Before placing in the file, mount each piece on brightly colored paper. The bulletin boards can be an eclectic selection of wellness topics, focus on a particular topic, or support a national health observance. Use the bulletin boards for tracking the status of ongoing wellness competitions, posting the calendar of events, and promoting the health promotion department itself. Rotate the subject matter monthly so the information does not become boring. Assign responsibility for maintaining the board to departmental volunteers. Volunteers check out the accordion file and other information to be posted. Ask volunteers to help find new material from newspapers, magazines, and other sources to add to the file.

- **In-house cable television**

Besides offering informational health and wellness videos throughout the day, look for do-it-yourself behavior modification videos. Such videos are usually structured like a multisession program offering information relevant to the various stages of a change process, assign activities to be accomplished before viewing the next segment of the tape, and include self-study material. Make the self-study material available for check-out to people wanting to participate in the program. Schedule the video to be viewed on the days corresponding to the "homework activities" assigned in the tape. On the viewing days, show the video more than once so employees can work a convenient time into their schedules and not miss a session. Post health promotion programming information and wellness tips on the cable system electronic marquee.

- **Adopt-a-class**

Offer graduates from past behavior modification programs the opportunity to "adopt" attendees of future programs. The graduates act as a support system for individuals or the entire class. Attendees are encouraged to call their adopter between sessions if they need advice, encouragement, and so on. Encourage the adopters to attend some or all of the classes to reinforce their own health goals as well as get to know the attendees. Encourage adopters to share their own experiences with changing their behavior in the class.

■ **Stressor programs**

Generic stress management programs serve a purpose for the severely stressed or those who cannot identify a source for their stress. But many people have specific reasons for being stressed. In these cases, programs designed to overcome the stressor itself are much more beneficial. Stressor programs reach individuals who have not self-identified as being stressed either because the problem has not reached a critical level or because stress management programs carry a stigma for them. Helping these people learn to deal with the stressor while it is only a minor problem may help them avoid becoming unduly stressed. Even for the severely stressed individuals, stressor programs would be a useful adjunct to a general stress management program. Their stress levels may automatically diminish as they learn to positively deal with their stressor. Typical stressors usually fall in one or more of the following areas: work, family, peer groups, finance, and communication skills. The more specific the information about the stressor, the more effective the program will be in meeting a group's need. To identify the stressors in a group's life, you must conduct a thorough needs assessment.

■ **Do-it-yourself tips for slides**

Illustrate a point or add a needed humorous touch to slide presentations with picture slides. The zoo offers a rich selection of animals to illustrate desirable or undesirable behaviors. A tortoise tells us to slow down; a giraffe eating leaves illustrates the value of a high-fiber diet to help us grow tall and run fast. Look for metaphors in life. Sailboats offer an excellent visual illustration of the calm waters of relaxation, the stormy seas of life, and the value of finding a sheltered harbor to escape the stresses of life. Adults respond to graphically displayed information better than raw data. Many computer graphics programs have the capability to make charts (pie charts, bar graphs, etc.).

There are many CD-ROM computer programs with hundreds of high-quality pictures on virtually every imaginable subject. There are some licensing constraints on how these pictures can be used, but in most cases, reproduction for use by the licensee in a classroom situation would be permitted. Some office supply companies carry a variety of slide and transparency pictures, cartoons, and motivational quotations for use in presentations, though these are more expensive. Typically, you purchase a set of slides or transparencies that fall under general subject matter categories, such as animals, boats, sunsets, medical.

It is possible to reproduce graphic and pictorial slides from a computer program by photographing the monitor screen in a darkened room with a macro lens. The cost for the slide program is merely the cost of printing the slide film. If you want to include picture slides in a computer-generated presentation, some film-developing companies will digitalize developed film for use on computers. The company sends a computer disk with the pictures. These disks can be integrated into many computer-generated presentation programs.

Many people prefer the self-study approach when addressing lifestyle problems. This is especially true in sensitive areas such as stress management and smoking cessation. Consider developing a slide presentation of a program, then reading the script onto an audiocassette, marking the points for advancing the slide to the next frame. Some organizations have the capability of making an automatic-advance cassette; but if that capability is not available, ringing a bell or simply saying "beep" into the microphone can inform the viewer when to advance the frame.

- **Do-it-yourself tips for transparencies**

Most copiers and many computer printers have the capability of making overhead transparencies from printed material. Anatomical pictures, cartoons, graphs, and print are just some of the possibilities when making transparencies. Some of the more advanced copiers can even make transparencies from 35mm slides. If a color printer is not available, black and white transparencies can be dressed up by highlighting main points or coloring graphs with overhead-projector pens.

Blank transparencies can be effective when group participation is desired. For example, in a stress management program, asking for signs of stress and writing them down for the group to see as they are provided is a valuable learning tool.

- **Do-it-yourself tips for flip charts**

One of the cheapest and simplest visual aids available is the flip chart. The speaker prepares a visual outline of his or her program prior to the class or writes down solicited input from the class. Broad-tipped markers may be all that is necessary for some programs. If a program is offered frequently, use a computer graphics program with a banner option. Use a "font" size of about two to three inches, print the desired outline, then tape the material onto the flip chart paper. This looks extremely professional and is very easy for the class to read.

9 Behavior Change Bingo

Everyone enjoys a game of bingo. Work that to your advantage. What group behavior are you trying to change? Can you measure it? If so, "Behavior Change Bingo" provides the group with motivation to maintain the desired change until it is integrated into their normal behavior.

Encouragement and approval from peers and coworkers is one of the strongest motivators within an organization. To achieve that type of support system, Behavior Change Bingo creates an environment in which the group, as well as the individual, has a vested interest in effecting long-term behavior change.

Goals

To reward accomplishment of a desired group behavior

To reinforce a desired behavior through peer pressure

Target audience

Employees within an organization of virtually any size

Process

- The value of this game is to motivate employees to monitor each other's behaviors and support the desired change.

  To encourage this, a prize of some value is necessary.

  Winners of the game should be given the prize immediately.

  All winners' names are placed into a lottery for an annual grand prize of even greater value.

- Identify areas where success or failure in achieving a desired behavior or goal can be readily identified:

  on-the-job accidents

  compliance with safety policies and use of safety equipment

  substance-abuse related accidents/offenses (on or off the job) seat-belt use

conformance with no-smoking policy

- Post the rules of the game and the behaviors that are considered an infraction to demonstrating the desired behavior change:

  any on-the-job accident

  off-the-job accidents/infractions reported through the police department or insurance company

  failure to use appropriate safety equipment/body mechanics reported by designated supervisors

  failure to use seat belts reported through police accident reports or by parking-lot guards/monitors

  failure during random drug testing

  smoking on the job or in designated no-smoking areas

- Provide all employees who wish to participate with a bingo card.
- Consider setting up some method to ensure each employee gets only one bingo card per game (such as a coding system).
- On the first day of the game and every day thereafter, a designated employee draws out a bingo number, which is then posted in some place that is easily accessible to all employees:

  marquee

  computer network bulletin board/E-mail

  public-address system

- Maintain a central game board, where employees can learn which numbers have been drawn in the current game.
- A new drawing occurs every day that no infraction of the rules has occurred.
- If an infraction of the rules does occur, all cards are pulled and the game starts over after a predetermined penalty period.

  Depending on the circumstances, describe the details of the infraction.

  Use of the person's name is usually not necessary.

- When an employee presents a winning card,

  verify the winning numbers;

post the winning numbers (employees usually like to see for themselves);

pull all cards and issue new ones (some companies use the same cards over and over, but if an employee wants to try a new card, he or she must return the old one);

- Start a new game the following day.

Variation

This strategy can be used in achieving production and deadline goals.

10 "I Caught You" Cards

Reward the small steps toward a positive lifestyle through "I Caught You" cards. At the same time, show employees that management recognizes and rewards healthy habits.

Acknowledging the small successes in changing behavior is as important as celebrating the big ones. In most work environments where career-oriented employees respect management, combining management recognition and approval with an ongoing, structured incentive program is highly effective in encouraging behavior change.

Goals

To encourage positive behaviors within the workforce

To raise management's awareness of health promotion goals

To show employees management's support of health promotion program

Target audience

Employee populations

Process

- Define desirable behaviors that can be observed or demonstrated within the workplace. Base desired behaviors on health promotion program goals and, where possible, management human resource goals. Examples:

  attainment of an established health goal: weight loss, tobacco-free

  personal growth: special training, college programs, completion of behavior modification course

  healthy eating: snacks, lunch breaks

  exercise: using the stairs instead of elevators, working out at lunch, walking during breaks

  workplace safety: practicing sound body mechanics, wearing safety equipment, asking for assistance when lifting or running large equipment conflict management

communication skills

teamwork

- Define supervisor responsibilities in participating in the incentive program, such as the number of cards to be disseminated within a set time frame (monthly, quarterly, etc.). Set up tracking systems to monitor whether supervisors give out all their cards each period and whether awarded cards are given for appropriate reasons. Health promotion staff should report on both elements in management meetings and encourage discussion when program goals are not met.
- Brief all supervisors on program and purpose of changing the identified behaviors. Provide written suggestions to assist supervisors in determining whether an action meets the criteria for a desirable behavior.
- Establish a process to ensure each supervisor receives his or her allotted cards at beginning of each period.
- Award of individual cards can be done informally, but supervisors should make an effort to pick a time when other employees are available to witness the event.
- Design of cards should include all necessary information on the incentive program, as well as a place for supervisors to write down this data:

  to whom the card is awarded

  date

  behavior observed
- Each card should have a defined value.
- Consider awarding a special incentive to the employee with the most accumulated cards in a period and/or a year.
- Ideally, the awarding of incentives should be conducted by senior management in a special setting, such as a luncheon or a general meeting of all employees.

Cross-Reference: Chapter 6, Bogus Bucks

11 Phone Clinics and Seminars

Are you responsible for health promotion programming at a multisite organization or for a geographically widespread target audience? If so, consider phone clinics. With the advent of telephone conferencing, this approach makes sense and is cost effective. What's more, large segments of underserved populations are now accessible.

Brochure, book, and video mail-outs are often the only recourse for reaching isolated audiences. Regional health educators encounter significant problems: (1) some audiences will still not be reached, especially in the case of enrolled patients in a health maintenance organization, (2) most program budgets cannot accommodate enough educators to be effective, and (3) regional programs underutilize specialized instructors or incur higher costs due to travel expenses. Phone clinics allow for centralization of health educators and optimal use of specialized educators and allow isolated audiences to participate in valuable personalized programs. All you need is access to telephone conference call services. A telephone with a no-hands speaker or headset is ideal but not essential.

Goals

To provide health and wellness programs to isolated customers

To efficiently utilize specialized health educators within a constrained budget

Target audience

Geographically separated audiences or audiences isolated by personal circumstance (inner city, full-time at home caregivers, disabled)

Process

- Since participants cannot see the facilitator, the instructor can script more of the program while still allowing spontaneity, group interaction, and question/answer sessions. It is best to limit each session to no more than an hour.
- Participants should be encouraged to dial into the program at the time for which they registered. However, since the same program can be offered throughout the day, participants could be given the opportunity to attend at alternative times

when a conflict arises. Since there are sometimes limitations on telephone line access, this option should be exercised only after discussion with the facilitator prior to the class.

Audiences that include stay-at-home mothers, the disabled, or adult caregivers can feel comfortable with participating in phone programs. They know they can hang up and deal with personal matters, then rejoin the program without being disruptive or embarrassed.

In some cases, employees calling from an office or work station can mute their phone and work while listening to the program.

- Mail paper copies of visual aids and any other program materials to participants prior to the program.
- If a support-group-type environment is desired, compile a short biography of all participants and include in participant mail-out packages. Encourage group bonding through icebreaker activities. Whole Person Associates' structured exercise manuals have many activities that could be modified for the telephone.
- Coordinate any physical assessments (cholesterol screening, blood pressure screening, percent body fat, etc.) with local health care provider networks. They conduct the required screenings and either provide the results to the participant or forward to the instructor/facilitator for use at the appropriate time in the program.
- More than one person speaking during a conference call will obliterate both voices. Everyone must identify him or herself by name and ask permission to speak. The facilitator determines who speaks and when.
- Marketing efforts should include

  mass mail-outs to target audiences, explaining operation of the phone clinic/seminar, program content, and time options from which to choose;

  a central point for telephone and/or mail-in registration.
- Consider the following variables when determining whether to hire full-time, part-time, or consultant health educators for managing the programs.

  Health educators do not have to be physically located in an office environment. Part-time or contract educators can even conduct the programs from their homes, representing an extra cost savings to the program.

  What is the anticipated demand for the program? How frequently will the program be offered? Since the program can be conducted by one instructor/

facilitator at a single location, it is possible to accommodate participant scheduling preferences and time zones by offering the same program at different times throughout the day, as well as on different days in the same week.

Are support services available to the health educator to minimize the administrative time? Depending on the program, the administrative burden could include

reviewing participant screening information;

maintaining a log with notes on each session (this is especially important in order to track issues raised during multiple session programs and/or to keep things organized when more than one program is being conducted in the same time frame);

forwarding facilitator notes on individual participants to physicians for inclusion in their personal records;

providing attendance records and other reporting documents to the central health promotion office;

conducting one-on-one consultation sessions with individual participants during and/or after the program(s).

- To determine which telephone conferencing option is best for your program, discuss your needs with internal organizational telephone support personnel as well as the local telephone company customer service department. They can then outline the pros and cons for each option. The most common methods for generating telephone conference calls are

  operator assisted—the operator calls all participants and links them together;

  caller linking—the facilitator/instructor dials each participant and links them together through a multiple capacity conference telephone;

  dedicated telephone conference lines—the operator gives the facilitator/instructor a special conference call number, and the instructor and the participants dial the number at the designated time.

Variation

Use a similar method to conduct inservices or staff meetings with geographically separated health educators and program volunteers.

12 Programming Decision Matrix

Keep target audiences and senior management happy when designing programs. Use this simple programming tool modified from proven quality improvement techniques. It will help you balance priorities and develop sound implementation strategies.

While a health promotion program cannot reasonably meet the needs and expectations of every customer, attempting to meet as many needs as possible is obviously a wise step. Any individual or group that in some way benefits from the success of the health promotion program is by definition a customer. Generally, it is corporate management that authorizes worksite wellness programs, yet their program expectations as customers are not carefully considered when developing program strategies. Incorporating customer criteria into marketing strategies encourages program enthusiasm and management support.

Goals

To develop programming strategies to meet the most significant needs and expectations of major customer segments

To focus programming resources on known areas of customer interest

Target audience

All types

Process

- Use the Programming Decision Matrix in the early stages of planning health promotion programs and services for an upcoming year.
- Based on needs assessment data, summarize important criteria for major customer groups. This is the information used in the decision matrix. A blank copy of the Programming Decision Matrix can be found at Figure 1. The matrix can be made larger or smaller depending on the complexity of customer criteria identified in the assessment process.

  At a minimum, this matrix helps ensure that programming strategies comply with management's expectations for the health promotion program while providing products and services that the employee customers desire.

- Figure 2 provides an example of the tool's use when comparing the hypothetical criteria of senior management against those of the organization employees.

  The needs assessment showed that the employees wanted health promotion programs to be fun, to learn their personal health risks, to have most wellness programs offered during the workday, and to have information on their health risks and other behavior problems kept private. In Figure 2, employee criteria are listed down the lefthand side of the matrix.

  Management's expectations for the health promotion program included that it would help the organization control health care costs and determine group health risks and that they would see an improvement in productivity and morale. In Figure 2, management criteria are listed across the top of the matrix.

- Program planners would develop at least one strategy for each of management's and employees' expectations in every box of the matrix. For example, the top lefthand box of Figure 2 calls for an incentive program to reduce use of the health care system. This strategy could include discouraging inappropriate use of the health care system through use of a self-care manual and holding a periodic raffle for a luxury vacation to employees who keep their health care costs for the year below a certain level. Obviously, a raffle for a vacation would be fun, thus meeting the employee's criterion; and the anticipated reduction of inappropriate use of the health care system would meet management's criterion of controlling health care costs.

  The second box on the bottom row of Figure 2 calls for eliminating references to individuals from group health risk-appraisal reports. This meets the employees' criteria for privacy of information, while still providing management with useful group information on health risks.

  The next step would be to further refine each strategy outlined in the matrix into specific programs, products, and services to be offered during the year.

- Program planners market the health promotion initiatives and activities developed from this exercise by illustrating how each strategy meets one or more criteria for employees.

- In presenting the proposal to management for funding and support, the health promotion manager emphasizes how the strategies meet management's criteria.

Cross-Reference: Chapter 14, Needs Assessments

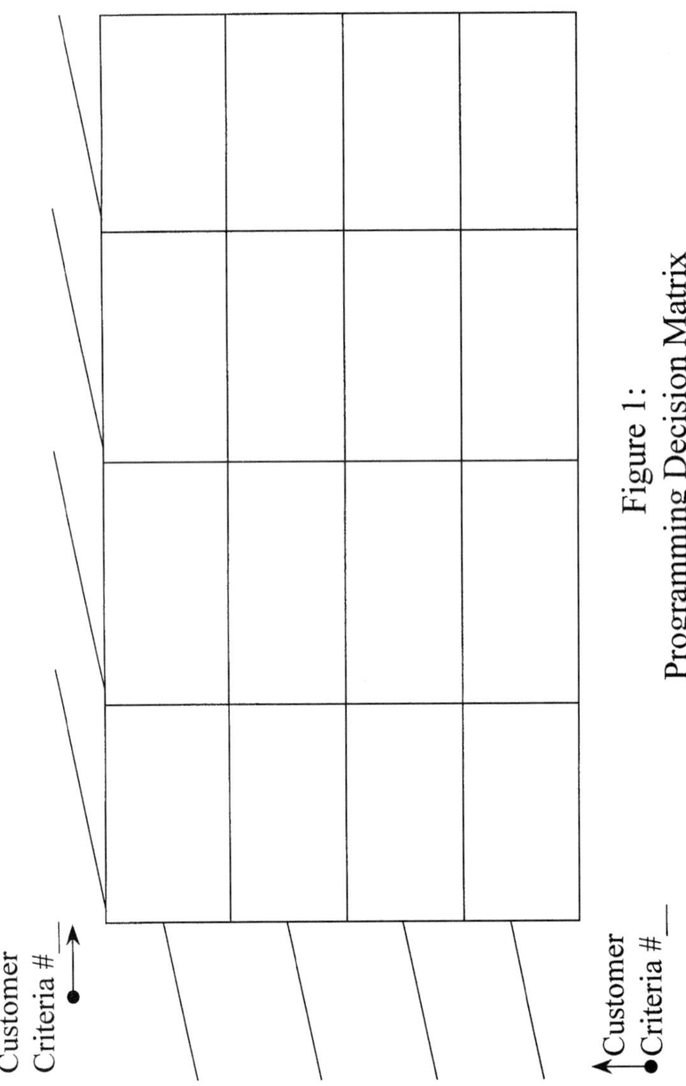

Figure 1:
Programming Decision Matrix

 (800) 247-6789

Management Criteria →

Employee Criteria ↑ \ Management Criteria →	Control Health Care Costs	Determine Group Health Risks	Improve productivity	Raise Morale
Make It Fun	Incentive program to reduce use of health care system	"Beat the Boss" assessment competitions. Prizes for best scores	Initiate health and safety competition with prizes	Fitness Day with Inter-Office Competition
Learn personal health risks	Lecture series based on HRA results	Health Risk Appraisal (HRA) Program with feedback loop	Develop special work hardening program based on HRA results	Include private fitness assessments in Fitness Day activities
Minimal Off-Duty Time	"Lunch and Learn" health risk programs	Health screen & counseling done during staff mtg.	Provide "comp" time for personnel attending off-duty	1-hour Tae Chi classes starting 1/2-hour before end of work
Ensure Privacy of Information	Compile group utilization reports only	"Sanitize" group HRA info so individuals can not be identified	Provide work stress programs but code records instead of names	Publicly recognize class successes (with permission)

Employee Criteria ↑

6

Figure 2:
Example Programming Decision Matrix

13 Journey to Wellness

Most health promotion competitions focus on aerobic exercise and little else. "Journey to Wellness" recognizes and rewards all aspects of balanced living. This easily maintained wellness competition relies heavily on self-responsibility, but provides ongoing incentives and sufficient oversight to encourage integrity and maintain motivation.

It is easy to be overwhelmed when beginning a personal wellness journey. Where do you start? Even wellness-oriented individuals can lose sight of the true goal of health promotion: achieving a healthy balance physically, mentally, socially, and spiritually in everything they do. Most health educators can think of someone who focused so much on one or two components of healthy living that it perhaps adversely affected some other important aspects of his or her life. Developing a program that places a defined value on each step toward a balanced lifestyle will greatly help all target audiences.

Goals

To encourage balanced healthy lifestyle

To increase participation and utilization of health promotion programs and services

Target audience

All types

Process

- "Journey to Wellness" is a race spanning an entire year. The race can be around a city, county, state, the United States, other countries, or the world. Starting and ending points are determined by the race organizers and can even be changed between races to help maintain interest.
- Draw a race course on a map. Maps of virtually any state, the United States, or other countries can be developed from computer clip art software programs or reproduced from clip art books found in any good bookstore.

  Design the course to run through landmarks of interest to participants. Landmarks help participants set short-term goals as well as achieve the ultimate goal of finishing the race.

Along the course map, place a series of mile-marker squares in increments reflecting appropriate mileage for the distance to be covered (e.g., 1 mile/square for a county or state, 4 miles/square for the United States or another country, 10 miles per square for an around-the-world competition).

- Participants earn "wellness miles" for accomplishing simple daily healthy activities. Determine what behaviors you wish to reward; define the frequency the behavior must be demonstrated; then allocate a mileage value to the behavior.

Examples of personal health activities (based on a cross-country course):

physical exam: one/year = 15 miles

blood pressure check: one/year = 2 miles

fitness test: one every four months = 10 miles/test

seat-belt use (all passengers): daily for one week = 2 miles/week

dental exam: maximum two/year = 5 miles/exam

vision exam: one/year = 5 miles

CPR certification/recertification: one/year = 3 miles

first-aid certification: one/year = 3 miles

cholesterol screening: one/year or per doctor's orders = 5 miles/test

quit smoking (only allowed to claim miles in each category once per year):

first month continuous = 25 miles

second month continuous = 25 miles

next four months = 10 miles/month

floss teeth: three times/week = 1 mile/week

donate blood: every two months = 5 miles/unit

Examples of nutrition activities (based on a cross-country course):

eating a nutritious well-balanced breakfast and drinking eight glasses of water, milk, or juice/day = 1/2 mile per day

weight control (behavior modification) program = 2 miles/class

weight control support group = 1 mile/meeting

yearly total weight loss = 2 miles/pound

reduction in percent body fat: maximum of one test per quarter = 4 miles per 1 percent body fat lost

Examples of mental health activities (based on a cross-country course):

- meditation/relaxation (tape or class setting): 30 minutes = 1 mile
- mental/emotional wellness seminar: 45 minutes = 1 mile
- books read (fiction or nonfiction): one book = 2 miles
- volunteering in an organizational or community activity: 60 minutes = 1 mile

Examples of aerobic activities (based on a cross-country course):

- fitness class: 60 minutes = 4 miles
- walking: 1 mile = 1 mile
- running: 1 mile = 1 mile
- swimming: 1/4 mile = 1 mile
- biking
  - outside: 2-1/2 miles = 1 mile
  - stationary: 10 minutes = 1 mile
- rowing machine: 10 minutes = 1 mile
- speed skating: 10 minutes = 1 mile
- cross-country ski machine: 10 minutes = 1 mile
- outdoor cross-country skiing: 60 minutes = 5 miles
- jump rope: 10 minutes = 1 mile
- stair-aerobic/stair machine: 10 minutes = 1 mile
- at home calisthenics: 30 minutes = 1 mile
- bonus points: extra 2 miles/week for aerobic exercise done three times in one week

Other physical activities (based on a cross-country course):

- racquetball, basketball, soccer: 60 minutes = 3 miles
- singles tennis: 60 minutes = 2 miles
- stair climb: 25 flights = 1 mile (may compile flights climbed over a period of days)
- stair descend: 50 flights = 1 mile (may compile flights descended over a period of days)

power volleyball: 60 minutes = 2 miles

rebounders/trampolines: 15 minutes = 1 mile

any martial art: 60 minutes = 2 miles

golf (walking): nine holes = 1-1/2 miles

Nautilus: 20–30 minutes = 2 miles

free or universal weights: 20–30 minutes = 2 miles

raking, mowing, or shoveling: 60 minutes = 2 miles

recreational biking: 30 minutes = 1 mile

recreational activities (60 minutes = 1 mile): softball, water-skiing, downhill skiing, doubles tennis, horseback riding, ice-skating, roller-skating, gardening, bowling, recreational volleyball

Other areas to consider (based on a cross-country course):

Recruiting a new member into the competition: 3 miles/person

Other wellness seminars: 45 minutes = 1 mile

- The competition can be structured for individuals or teams.
- Each participant is given these tools:

  set of rules for "Journey to Wellness"

  conversion chart that reflects healthy activities and the miles awarded to each activity

  diary to track their activities ("Journey to Wellness" is played on the honor system; the diary provides competition organizers a method to validate miles earned.)

  race course map to fill out with accrued miles
- To maintain motivation, set landmarks along the course where smaller incentives are awarded. These smaller incentives can either be picked up at any time or be awarded publicly at a monthly group recognition event.
- Set the annual deadline for reaching the finishing mile marker. Participants reaching the finish line by that point become eligible for a grand prize drawing.
- A new competition for the next year can be immediately started after the deadline for the current year's competition has been reached. Distribute a new map with appropriate mile markers at that time.

14 Needs Assessment

In order to deliver a health message that is understood and accepted, health promotion managers must appreciate the realities and life challenges faced by their target audiences. Health-risk appraisals do not provide that kind of information. This chapter defines the customer information you MUST know and outlines some strategies for gaining it.

The usefulness of group information compiled in health risk appraisals is limited without insights into group behaviors contributing to the risk factors, external and internal obstacles to changing customers' negative behavior, the customers' level of motivation to change, and the perceived value of the health promotion program. Generic "one-size-fits-all" health promotion programming will never have the impact of customized information or services.

Goals

To gain insights into the cultural and life experiences of a target audience

To design health promotion products and services that best meet customer expectations and needs

Target audience

All types

Process

- The needs assessment process is crucial to program success. Use the information to ensure that senior management's goals for the health promotion program are being addressed;

  By incorporating management's priorities into programming strategies, health promotion managers help secure their program's long-term survival against the rise and fall of changing organization priorities.

  If the assessment identifies unrealistic management goals for the program, include strategies for educating management in the programming planning process.

determine the best times, days, and locations to offer programs to major customer segments;

Compare this information against any days or times identified by management as critical times effecting organizational productivity.

Look for windows of opportunity to satisfy both customers.

discover any obstacles to attending programs, such as transportation problems or child care, that can be addressed;

purchase/develop education and awareness materials to meet reading, language, and accessibility limitations;

develop specific intervention and awareness strategies based on customer groups' current readiness to change;

develop marketing strategies using resources and methods identified by target audiences:

informal target-audience leaders who can help influence participation in health promotion initiatives

places where the target audience congregates that can be used to disseminate information

economical and effective methods to get written materials to the home or work.

address significant biases or problems that impede customer participation in programs. Look at programs with the eyes of the audience:

Are there religious or cultural influences that affect a behavior? For instance, many Native Americans use tobacco in their religious ceremonies. A message to quit smoking without considering their religious beliefs would be unpopular.

Is there anything in the material, the environment, or the instructor that is intimidating or sends a negative message? For instance, older or significantly overweight customers may view high-energy aerobics classes taught by young, athletic aerobics instructors as being beyond their capability or embarrassing.

Is the environment of the audience a problem? Can inner-city audiences reach a program safely? Can single parents afford child care?

- While health promotion customers include anyone directly benefiting from program services, it is also wise to include in the assessment process people or departments that indirectly benefit from these services. They can provide insights into their own health promotion needs, as well as identify issues impacting on other target audiences influenced by them. This includes the following:

employer groups: chief executive officer, departmental supervisors, board of directors, shift workers, the different staff found at multisite organizations, human resources, and traveling staff (e.g., salespeople)

schools/colleges: teachers, students (by demographics), nonacademic staff, parents/PTA, school board, alumni

hospitals/clinics: medical staff, inpatients, outpatients, nonmedical staff (administrative, volunteers)

community: community laymen (by demographics), local businesses, area nonprofit agencies (e.g., United Way), local political leaders, government agencies (e.g., public health department)

- Further identify these customer categories by age, gender, ethnicity, education, and income.
- Issues such as language differences, marital status, presence of children, inner-city versus urban dwellers, and religion may be of concern to some program planners.
- Once customer categories have been defined, conduct an assessment of what each group's health promotion needs are and how best to present the desired information. To gather information on individual and group health risks, you have a wealth of commercial health-risk assessments from which to choose; but a good "needs" assessment tool is harder to find. It may be necessary to design a tool that is specific to your program's needs.
- In most cases, more than one assessment approach will be needed:

  it may be best for a senior representative (or advocate) of the health promotion department to personally survey the organization's senior management and interview middle managers about their concerns privately;

  mail-out surveys may be the only option for multisite organizations or traveling employees;

  conducting group health-risk appraisals and needs assessments may be best for students, shift workers, and departmental employees.
- Whatever the assessment process, gain as much of the following customer information as possible:

  the demographic data outlined above

behavioral and genetic health risks

desired health education program components

personal health/quality of life priorities

best program times, days, locations, length, etc.

organizational health/productivity goals

past participation in health education programs

readiness to improve on health risks

people/places/forums to market programs

perceptions/biases concerning health

challenges to successful program participation, self-responsibility, prevention programs: language, work, family responsibilities, etc.

resources customer can contribute: time, money, equipment, facility, etc.

desired format of services rendered: video, lecture, pamphlets, newsletters, self-study, etc.

In assessment of middle and senior managers, additional information concerning their concerns about the impact of the health promotion program on organizational productivity, goals, and objectives will help assure program planners that management will not undermine their efforts.

- When designing a needs assessment tool, ask the following questions:

  How well do current health promotion programs and services meet their needs?

  If they do not participate in current health promotion programs, why?

  What written information on specific topics do they desire?

  What health promotion subjects do they desire?

  What needs to happen for them to change a behavior?

  What is their biggest source of stress?

  What health evaluation do they most desire?

  What is their primary source for finding out what is happening in their community or work?

  If they are interested in helping support the health promotion program, what conditions for volunteering must exist?

Cross-Reference: Chapter 5, Focus Groups; Chapter 12, Programming Decision Matrix

15 Databases

Just a few reasons for tracking program attendees and other interested personnel include doing target marketing, conducting follow-ups, and identifying volunteers to help in program activities. This chapter includes tips on high- and low-tech strategies for maintaining databases and putting them to their best use.

The more effectively a health promotion manager manipulates information about customers, support personnel, and resources, the more efficiently and economically he or she can focus valuable resources for marketing and program development.

A computer with a spreadsheet program will enable the health promotion manager to do the strategies outlined below. If the health promotion manager is not skilled in operating a computer, support from someone with those skills will be necessary. A simple low-tech suggestion is provided for managers without access to a computer, but they will be restricted in their ability to accomplish some of the suggestions.

Goals

To track participation and progress of individuals towards their health goals

To efficiently target audiences for specific marketing initiatives

To identify potential resources for program support

To provide easily accessible and accurate information on the health promotion program

Target audience

All types

Process

- It is not the intent of this chapter to teach the health promotion manager how to use a computer database. The applications computer databases can bring to a health promotion program are just the tip of the iceberg. Computers are an invaluable ally. Take advantage of the many avenues to learn about computers and computer programs. Many organizations offer free classes to their employees. Adult education programs are available in most communities.

- Computer databases can be developed from most basic spreadsheet programs. Lotus and Excel are two popular software programs. Examples of sources for spreadsheet information and the uses they can be put to:

  individual counseling sessions: tracking progress towards health goals, sending out topical information or marketing pieces for upcoming programs based on interests identified during the counseling session, flagging client records for scheduling follow-up sessions

  needs assessments: sending out topical information or marketing pieces for upcoming programs based on needs assessment requests

  health-risk appraisals and health evaluations: tracking changes in individual health risks (smoking, activity levels, stress levels, etc.) and health screening results (cholesterol, blood sugar, blood pressure, etc.); targeting mail-outs of handouts and program announcements based on identified health risks; notifying customers for follow-ups on health screenings; manipulating information to determine specific target-audience risks

  program registration and attendance records: monitoring program utilization based on target audiences, preparing utilization reports

  administrative tracking of assets such as speakers, volunteers, equipment, facilities

- Although somewhat limited in its value, one effective method for maintaining a database without a computer is a simple card file.

  For targeted mail-outs, place a 3 x 5 card with name, phone number, address, and the type of programs or information to send customers in a card file broken down by topic (stress, fitness, nutrition, etc.).

  To identify resources for program support, maintain a file for hard assets such as facility, chairs and tables, audiovisual equipment. Keep another file for speakers and other support personnel with their names, phone numbers, relevant biographical information, and the types of programs or support expertise they can provide. If the number of speakers and support personnel is significant, it is probably wise to file their information under program categories (stress, fitness, nutrition, etc.) even if it means making more than one card for individuals who support more than one type of program.

- A strategy for managing follow-ups without a computer requires an accordion file. During an appointment or while attending a class, participants fill out envelopes with their mailing addresses. The participant or health promotion staff place necessary follow-up materials in the envelope. The stamped and sealed envelope is then put in the accordion file under the month or week the document is to be mailed out. Mark mail-out days on a calendar. On the appropriate days, the health promotion manager, pulls whatever envelopes are in the accordion file for that period and puts them in the mail.

Cross-Reference: Chapter 5, Focus Groups; Chapter 14, Needs Assessment

16 Health Promotion Committees

A successful health promotion program requires top to bottom involvement of major target audiences and seeks out potential programming partners. Learn how to effectively structure and manage health promotion committees and how to use subcommittees to enhance efficiency and encourage involvement of key players.

It is much easier to integrate wellness concepts into the fabric of an organization or community when representatives of the customers, as well as other departments or agencies with a vested interest in the health, well-being, and quality of life of the customers, can provide the health promotion staff with ongoing input. This input includes customer involvement in program planning, development, and evaluation. A governing body that provides a structure for action and discussion of relevant issues is essential.

Goals

To provide a forum for exchanging information with target audiences

To improve program efficiency through a cooperative working relationship with individuals and agencies impacting on target-audience well-being

To provide a forum for evaluating the impact of the health promotion program

Target audience

All types

Process

- The first step in forming a health promotion committee is one of the most important. Present the committee concept to the most senior level of management possible and solicit their support. Request the following support:

  a senior management representative on the committee

  letters of appointment for all other members generated under the signature of a senior official, preferably the chief executive officer or equivalent

  This official backing will generate the necessary cooperation and support as the committee becomes a reality.

- Ideally, members of the committee should be volunteers, although it may be necessary to appoint certain members by virtue of their position and potential contribution to the committee. Depending on the type of program, consider requesting representatives from the following areas:

  medical: nurse, doctor, physician assistant, dietitian, social worker, mental health specialist

  eating facilities frequented by target audience: managers of the cafeteria, snack bar, or vending machines

  large customer segments: union, blue-collar and white-collar workers, spouses, ethnic or cultural groups, retiree organizations

  agencies with insights into personal issues relevant to the customers: human resources department, employee assistance department, chaplains

  youth organizations: YMCA, schools, day-care centers

  agencies with a health education responsibility that may be useful to your health promotion program goals: United Way, department of public health

- Depending on the scope of the health promotion program, committee membership could become too large and unwieldy to be effective. In such situations, consider forming subcommittees charged with working issues related to specific components of wellness or program management. These subcommittees function as the working arm of the central health promotion committee and report their activities to it. The following are only a few ideas to consider for subcommittees:

  a component of health promotion: nutrition, fitness, tobacco deglamorization

  marketing and information dissemination to target audiences: produces calendars, provides briefings, updates formal and informal leaders, develops marketing strategies

  special events, such as health fairs, fitness events, and special programs: handles the logistics of setting up the program, including obtaining equipment, volunteers, and speakers

  humor: develops ideas to integrate into other programs and initiatives to make the programs more fun

  Assign representatives whose focus is confined to a single aspect of wellness to the appropriate subcommittee. For instance, representatives from a cafeteria or snack bar might be better utilized in a subcommittee tasked with addressing the nutrition needs of a group. The chairperson of each subcommittee sits on the central health promotion committee and reports on his or her subcommittee actions and recommendations.

Before creating new subcommittees, find out if there are already existing committees or organizational meetings that have many of the members who would logically sit on your proposed subcommittee. Request that this body assume responsibility for the subcommittee activity as part of the function of their committee/meeting. If there is someone missing from the committee, arrange with the chairperson to schedule the health promotion component at a specific time, then invite the missing people to show up for that time period.

- Once the membership and committee/subcommittee structure is established, the next step is to write a charter that defines the purpose of the committee. A well-written charter keeps the membership focused. The charter should be short and concise and easily accessible for each meeting. If discussion appears to be drifting off on a tangent, the chairperson asks everyone to refer to the charter. If it is agreed the topic does not support the charter, it is dropped. The charter should address these factors:

  community assessments: who will do it, how will it be done, and what will be done with the information

  a process to review existing programs and develop new programs/initiatives

  monitoring of the health/wellness environment of the community

  a forum for disseminating health information to the community

  measurement of program impact through trend analysis of indicators such as program metrics, surveys, screenings, critiques, follow-ups, etc.

- The next step is to develop the goals and objectives for the committee. It is crucial that the goals and objectives be developed by the committee and not spoon-fed to them by the health promotion staff. It is difficult to be committed to something when the individual has not had any input into the process. Require each committee member to set his or her own goals and objectives in support of the committee's and to present them for review.

  It is appropriate for the health promotion staff to present the results of surveys, assessments, group reports on health-risk appraisals and other wellness evaluations, and on program success rates and failures; but the committee must decide the priorities based on the information.

- Once the goals and objectives have been set, establish meaningful metrics on how the committee can track their progress towards accomplishment. The metrics should reflect what is important to the group, be realistic and within the control of the group, and be tracked as an ongoing agenda item for each meeting. An alternative to tracking the metrics in the central committee is to form a subcommittee to fill this function.
- It is easy for a committee to start losing their enthusiasm once the excitement of starting something new has worn off. The health promotion manager faces a significant challenge in combating this apathy. Instilling in the committee members a strong sense of ownership will help them maintain their competitive edge and excitement.

  Assign committee responsibilities to each member and hold them accountable for their actions. The letters of appointment or supporting policies should outline each member's responsibilities. The member or an informed representative must attend all meetings. Take action when a member does not fulfill his or her responsibilities.

  Recognize each member's contributions. Thank them frequently. Talk about their activities in public forums. Solicit quotes from members for wellness articles. Send letters to their supervisors complimenting them on their contributions. Bring a surprise treat to the meeting for no reason. Award certificates of accomplishment. Basically, let the committee members know that their services are valued.

  Consider a semiannual one-to-three-day retreat for the committee members, where they review their accomplishments, do some strategic planning, experience their own health and wellness evaluations, and are offered special programs aimed at their own personal needs, as well as provided with information they can use in their role as a committee member.

  The activities and decisions of the committee should be a group decision. The health promotion manager suggests alternatives and keeps the group focused, but must be willing to comply with a decision that may not be totally in keeping with his or her opinion. If the perception becomes that the health promotion staff will do what they want anyway, the group loses motivation and enthusiasm.

- One of the quickest ways to kill motivation and enthusiasm is to have an inefficiently run committee. While there are many aspects to efficient committee management, one of the most significant components is developing and following a well thought out agenda:

  get the agenda into the committee members' hands at least three to five workdays before the meeting;

  highlight items for each member who has responsibility to report on its status;

  discuss with individual members important or sensitive issues before the meeting to ensure that they are done and minimize potentially embarrassing situations;

  be supportive to members with open items but keep the responsibility for accomplishing the assignment on them. Advise them and provide ideas on how to accomplish their assignment, but hold them accountable;

  consider a pre-agenda, which would be sent out about two weeks before the agenda. Besides reminding the members to take action on their open items, the pre-agenda solicits input for "new business" on the final agenda;

  to keep the committee focused on their priorities, set the agenda around the committee's goals. Ask what is being done to accomplish the goals and identify any problem areas;

  if the most senior official of the organization does not personally sit on the committee, have the agenda reflect the person as an "ex-officio" member and the minutes reflect that a copy goes to him or her. Perhaps the committee can periodically meet as a group with senior management.

- Some form of written record of the committee's activities should be maintained.

  Be brief, but include sufficient information for the uninformed reader to understand the issues and the action taken. The minutes should reflect the names of all members, their organization, and whether they were present or represented.

  Consider the minutes of the committee as a communication tool and a record of events. It is acceptable to include documents as attachments rather than rewriting them into the body of the minutes. Any reference to documents, assessments, letters, articles, etc., made in the committee should be marked and attached to the committee minutes.

Any identified problems should be tracked to resolution. Items should not be closed prematurely if some aspect of the issue has not been resolved/accomplished. The only exception to this would be if, after discussion, the committee felt nothing could be done to resolve the issue. The reasons for lack of resolution should be documented prior to closure.

Health Fairs

24 **Parenting Fairs** 95

A health fair focusing on parenting issues provides services, customized health screenings, information booths, displays, demonstrations, and lectures of specific interest. Fair organizers are reminded to consider the unique parenting needs of men as well as women.

25 **Men's/Women's Fairs** 98

A health fair targeting gender-specific issues and health needs offers customized health screenings, information booths, displays, demonstrations, and lectures of specific interest.

26 **Focused Health Fairs** 101

This fair targets a specific category or component of health rather than all areas. Topic-related screenings, information booths, displays, demonstrations, and lectures are provided with a depth that would be difficult in more broad-based fairs. The focus remains on how to achieve optimum health in the targeted area.

17 Quick Tips

Some techniques fit into many types of programs. Try these quick tips with any of the fairs in this section or with your own programs.

■ **Partnering to increase attendance and participation**
When there is flexibility as to the date of a health fair, attempt to tie it to another event that would draw the same target audience. Partner with other health and community agencies that would also benefit from expanded marketing. For instance, the American Red Cross can be very open to offering blood drives in conjunction with another event. Other partnering ideas: arts and crafts fairs to draw senior citizens and women, safety programs put on by police and fire departments to attract parents and kids, pediatric clinics to expand annual school physicals into a children's health fair, and antique car shows to attract men.

■ **Incentives to increase attendance and participation**
Approach product vendors to help sponsor the fair through offering prizes relevant to the health fair focus: blood-glucose monitors at diabetic fairs, blood-pressure monitors at a senior citizen fair, child car seat at a parenting fair, and so on. Local corporate sponsors such as medical equipment supply stores, pharmacies, supermarkets, care centers for kids or senior citizens, health food stores, and restaurants may be equally enthusiastic. Either type of corporate sponsor is always looking for opportunities to gain name recognition among their target audiences. They will expect to see their name used in marketing, displayed during the fair, and included in any other way possible. Use these incentives in hourly drawings for anyone present in the fair area. Another strategy is to give incentives to anyone who visits all the health fair booths and/or receives a required combination of health screenings. This strategy requires a form to be filled out at each booth (see below) to prove the visits occurred. Also vendors can provide small incentives for booth prizes, such as pens, buttons, and refrigerator magnets, with their company logo imprinted.

■ **Coordinating speakers and demonstrations**
The best health fairs offer speakers and demonstrations in conjunction with other more traditional screening and awareness activities. Place flyers of all speakers and their presentation topics at every fair booth. Highlight the programs that relate to the booth topic. Instruct the staff at each booth to encourage visitors to see the

appropriate programs for more information. For instance, a blood-pressure screening booth should make a point of encouraging people with an elevated blood pressure to attend a scheduled program on coronary artery risks. Similarly, instruct speakers or demonstrators to encourage attendees at their programs to visit booths featuring services or information relating to their topic.

■ **Involving support groups and the community**

United Way agencies and other nonprofit support groups are eager for exposure to attract support and reach their target audiences. Even organizational health fairs should invite agencies to participate whose focus is related to a topic or audience reached by their fair. Offer them booth space to promote their organization. Ask for support with screenings, manning, traffic control, demonstrations, equipment, speakers, or panel discussions. In return, provide them with information on the numbers of participants. This is important to nonprofit agencies in gaining funding. Invite community agencies that offer services to the target audience. The police, fire departments, paramedic departments, community hospitals, department of public health, and Social Security and Medicare/Medicaid offices have valuable information to share. Even libraries may be interested in developing a display of books on topics relevant to the focus of the health fair.

■ **Use of videos and displays**

As the floor plan for the health fair is developed, consider where large groups are expected to be doing a lot of standing and waiting. These are the ideal locations to set up short videos and displays. Groups waiting for a blood-pressure check, blood-glucose test, or body-fat measurement are ideal examples. Set up VCRs and displays in the logical area where the traffic pattern will require these audiences to wait their turn. Short videos—five or ten minutes—are the best for this scenario. If possible, copy short videos onto one long-running tape to avoid constant changing. It is a good idea to post a sign over the VCR, listing the title or subject matter of the video. This is especially true if more than one video is being shown. If long videos are to be shown, set up the VCR in a more isolated area with chairs.

Each display should have one high-impact message. There are some excellent commercial displays available, but don't be afraid to make your own. Many interesting "info-bites" that can be found in wellness newsletters and articles could be graphically illustrated. For instance, with one or two cartoons or pictures and large colorful letters, a great display in a nutrition health fair could be made on how to absorb as much iron as possible from a meal or supplement. (Avoid tea, bran, or calcium within two to four hours before or after the meal or supplement. Eat or drink a vitamin-C food when taking the iron product to absorb more iron—but don't drink calcium-fortified orange juice.)

- **Information and activity booths**

Many times health fair information booths do not attract as much attention as a screening booth. People like to be involved: touching, feeling, doing. Typically, awareness information is given to participants verbally or in handouts. Add a relevant activity to information booths. Make use of the many commercial products available: larger-than-life mouth models to show the effects of oral tobacco; plastic fetuses in a bottle that blow smoky bubbles out their mouths, discoloring their "amniotic" fluid, to illustrate the hazards of smoking during pregnancy; computerized self-assessment software programs; and much more. But again, don't be afraid to develop a "homemade" activity booth. Modify old carnival games. For instance, pitch balls at a stack of cigarette packs or beer cans, toss darts at balloons containing grocery store coupons inside at a nutrition booth. The prizes do not have to be large: a pen, a toy, coupons, a refrigerator magnet, and the like.

- **Forms**

Give everyone a map of the health fair, showing location of booths and displays and a schedule of speakers/demonstrations, and a form with all the screening booths listed on it. This form should include a place to list each screening, the results, and a recommendation (diet, activity, see a doctor, etc.). Booth volunteers fill out the form at each station. An incentive is given to return the completed form to a table of volunteers before leaving the health fair (see "Tracking").

- **Tracking**

Set up a reception desk at the entrance to the health fair. Everyone entering must provide a name, address, and (optional) phone number. An incentive is given to return the completed form before leaving the fair. The reception desk volunteers review the form for any critical abnormals, make sure the participants understand their instructions, and document any relevant information for internal health promotion program statistics (numbers attended, booths visited, abnormals, etc.). This documentation can be coordinated with the demographic information gathered on attendees when they registered or listed in a simple column where volunteers place checks under the appropriate categories being tracked. A follow-up phone call to participants with abnormal screening results may be appropriate to ensure that action has been taken or help them access the necessary follow-up care.

18 Chronic Disease/Disability Fairs

Encouraging maximum independence and self-responsibility in populations with chronic diseases or disabilities is the goal of every health professional. Fairs that target the health needs of these populations and provide strategies to optimize quality of life are popular, as well as a sound health care management strategy.

The more independence people with chronic disease conditions and disabilities can exercise, the less they draw on costly community and health care services. Yet many people in these target audiences are unaware of the wide variety of support products and programs available to them. Disease and disability fairs can be the first step to open these doors.

Goals

To provide screening and information services that enable target audiences to optimize physical and emotional resources

To evaluate target audiences to determine future health and wellness programming needs

Target audience

Audiences with physical or mental challenges, selected by identified common needs and demographics

Process

- Make sure everything at your health fair is accessible and adapted to attendees with disabilities.
- Ideas for partnering:

  nonprofit organizations related to illness or condition—e.g., Special Olympics, American Diabetic Association, Arthritis Foundation, Asthma and Allergy Foundation of America, American Council of the Blind, American Paralysis Association

  health care providers specializing in the care of target audiences

- Ideas for activities:

  offer audience-specific health-risk appraisals and needs assessments. Besides providing feedback to each person being screened, use the group reports for determining future programming strategies.

  Have specialists and technicians check wheelchairs, prosthetics, and other support equipment used by people with disabilities and chronic diseases, to ensure good working order and to repair problems before they become major.

  Attempt to have volunteers with the same disabilities helping at the fair. It is especially important to have translators to assist hearing-impaired audiences in presentations and counseling.

  Hold fitness competitions based on disability: wheelchair races, foot races for the visually handicapped with a sighted guide or for runners with prosthetics, etc.

- Ideas for presentations and demonstrations:

  panels of people with the highlighted disease/disability discussing their strategies to maintain independence, a positive outlook, and relationships

  doctors discussing new advances in treatment

  exercise demonstrations designed for specific disabilities or special needs

  complementary medicine experts providing objective discussion of the pros and cons of less traditional remedies and treatments

  demonstration of self-help computer software programs and opportunities for attendees to use them

  demonstrations of equipment that may be useful to audiences with the highlighted disease or disability

  dogs and other animals trained to assist those with disabilities

  weight management issues relevant to the population

  strategies for modifying the home (with and without contractors) for a highlighted disability

- Ideas for screenings:

  for those with asthma or emphysema: lung capacity

  for people who use wheelchairs or have prosthetics: skin integrity, strength and flexibility for those with diabetes: blood glucose, foot and skin checks, dental, eye exams, blood pressure

- Ideas for information/awareness booths:

  pharmacies with information on therapeutic drugs

  nonprofit organizations related to illness or condition

  community support groups

  schools/institutions for training or rehabilitation of children and adults with disabilities or diseases

  nutrition consultants

  companies with products or services relevant to disease or disability

- Ideas for displays:

  displays/sales of self-help books related to the disease or condition

  information on national schools and clinics specializing in treatment of the disease or condition

  pictures and biographies of famous/successful people with the disease or disability

  appropriate aids for independence

    large-grip utensils and other adapted household items

    wheelchairs and accessories for them

    home oxygen systems

    monitoring units: diabetes, cholesterol, heart rate

    air purification systems for respiratory illnesses

    prosthetics

    telephones, doorbells, televisions, computers, and the like for people with vision or hearing impairments

Cross-Reference: Chapter 17, Quick Tips; Section 8, Resources

19 Ethnically and Culturally Oriented Fairs

In any given population, there are often small homogenous subgroups with statistically greater health risks than the general population; yet frequently these same groups are the least inclined to participate in wellness programs. Ethnic or culturally oriented health fairs are a major strategy to reach these underserved audiences.

It is not uncommon for audiences with strong cultural ties to be somewhat isolated from the general population. This isolation can be self-imposed or a result of language differences, cultural biases, and fear of the unknown. This isolation limits the audience's access to the health care system. Health problems may go untreated until they are in the advanced stages, and totally preventable illnesses run rampant. For the most part, health fairs for these audiences provide the same basic health services as a traditional fair, but are often the first exposure to American medicine. Consequently, this experience must be positive and packaged to appeal to the unique needs of each group.

Goals

To provide screening and information services to a target audience not reached adequately by traditional health and wellness programming

To gather target audience metrics concerning future health and wellness needs

Target audience

Audiences with a strong cultural or ethnic connection who are selected by identified common needs and demographics

Process

- Ideas for partnering:

  local political and community organizations dedicated to advancing issues and promoting causes relevant to the culture/ethnic group

  primary religious groups of the audience

  informal leaders within the target audience

- Ideas for activities:

  Health-risk appraisals and needs assessments: Besides providing feedback to each person being screened, use the group reports for determining future programming strategies

- Have as many volunteers as possible with the same background as the target audience. It is especially important to have an adequate number of volunteers to help orient and translate for attendees with limited English-speaking ability.

  It is important to note that many ethnic and cultural groups are not homogeneous. As you plan, consider the subgroups within populations. For instance:

  Hispanics: groups such as Mexicans, Puerto Ricans, Cubans, etc., have their own cultures.

  Asians and Pacific Islanders: this group comprises more than twenty different population groups and speak more than fifty languages and dialects

  Native Americans: this group includes many nations (tribes), with different languages and cultures.

- All written material should be in English and the primary language of the audience. Prior to the fair ask a volunteer who speaks the second language to read all materials not only to ensure appropriate content, but to look for references that may be misinterpreted due to cultural differences.

- Ideas for presentations and demonstrations:

  music, food, arts and crafts relevant to the audience to help draw in this group and make them feel comfortable

  informal and formal leaders of this group to provide opening remarks and periodic commentary on the importance of topics being presented

- Ideas for screening: In addition to the expected screenings for the audience's age and sex, identify risks specific to the target audience. A good source for identifying these risks is the goals set forth in Healthy People 2000, which highlights risk factors based on ethnic/cultural background. Examples of a few risks:

  African: sickle-cell anemia, high blood pressure, HIV

  Asian: growth retardation, hepatitis B

  Latin American: HIV

When language is a consideration, offer language screenings and referrals to self-help groups working in the necessary languages.

- Ideas for information/awareness booths:

  mentor programs for non-English-speaking adults and children: help in learning to read and speak English as well as other aspects of adapting to American life

  cultural/ethnic special interest groups

  local doctors, clinics, and health care agencies who wish to introduce themselves to this audience

- Ideas for displays (all in the audience's primary language):

  relevant health statistics found in Healthy People 2000 and sources for more information or help; for instance:

  41–62 percent of American Indian youth use marijuana, compared to 28–50 percent of the general population (note: there is significant tribal variability);

  in 1987, the lung cancer rate among African Americans was 38.5 per 100,000 and in 1992, 39.3 per 100,000; in the general population, rates have declined;

  in 1987, the chronic obstructive pulmonary disease (COPD) rate in African Americans was 18.9 per 100,000 and in 1992, 19.9 per 100,000;

  the five major causes of early death for American Alaskan Indians are unintentional injuries, cirrhosis, homicide, pneumonia, and the complications of diabetes;

  the incidence of diabetes in American Indians is 230 percent higher than in the general population; this is linked to adoption of the majority-culture diet and a significantly higher incidence of obesity.

  health posters written in the primary language

Cross-Reference: Any of the health fair chapters in this group are relevant to this chapter, as well. It is important to integrate the recommendations in this chapter into the strategies mentioned in the other chapters to attract the audience. Also, refer to Section 8 for information on how to attain a copy of Healthy People 2000.

20 Preschool Fairs

Geared toward high-energy and experiential activities, preschool health fairs expose children to health concepts, laying the groundwork for evolving attitudes and behaviors. This chapter provides ideas for learning experiences for the child and recommends health screenings and other services for consideration when planning this type of health fair.

Meeting the health and wellness needs of children is notoriously difficult. The challenges in first getting their attention, then maintaining their interest are very real, but can be overcome if you remember two important principles of wellness programming: (1) keep it fun; (2) customize to the age and understanding of the audience.

Goals

To introduce children to wellness concepts via a series of high energy, entertaining events

To provide child health screenings and safety services for parents

Target audience

Children age 3–5

Process

- Ideas for activities:

  healthy snacks: offer these to the kids, then give the parents recipes of the snacks their kids like.

  ball toss at a food pyramid or bull's-eye target: tape pictures of healthy foods on the inside of the target and unhealthy foods/snacks on the outside.

  "What's in me?": prior to the fair, buy a child-sized stuffed animal and remove the stuffing. Make cloth organs for the animal and place inside. Seal the abdomen with velcro. The kids take turns reaching inside the animal, pulling out the organ, and discussing its function with the facilitator.

Teddy bear clinic: children bring their teddy bear to a doctor/nurse for a checkup. The child helps the teddy bear not be scared by letting the health care provider demonstrate how it is done on him or her.

Kidnapping prevention program: fingerprinting and videotaping

"Where do germs come from?": Place a different color of glitter in a series of bowls. Each child places a hand in a different bowl. Encourage the children to play together for a few minutes. Then bring them together to find signs of the glitter on each other and around the room. Explain that germs are transmitted the same way, which is why we should all wash our hands.

- Ideas for presentations and demonstrations:

  wellness stories read or told by a storyteller

  wellness puppet shows on topics such as going to bed on time, sharing, eating right, personal hygiene, reasons why people are different physically and mentally

  police/fire department/ambulance service/med-flight teams show children the inside of police car/fire truck/ambulance/helicopter

  police dog demonstration

  practice 911 calls: If possible, ask a police officer to teach the kids what "911" is for and to place a special practice call into the emergency response system. Use a speaker phone so all the children can hear the conversation. If that is not possible, use a real phone for the child to dial 911 and have a facilitator play the role of the operator on another phone in the room.

- Suggested screenings:

  speech

  immunization

  scoliosis

  posture

  lead

  height/weight

  dental

  speech

  respiratory

TB

HIV (for high-risk groups)

sickle-cell anemia (children of African and Mediterranean heritage)

Cross-Reference: Chapter 17, Quick Tips; Chapter 21, Elementary School Fairs; Chapter 43, Quick Tips

21 Elementary School Fairs

Elementary-age students enjoy a carnival-like health fair where they can participate with appropriate adult supervision independent from their parents/caregivers. Health screenings, parenting topics, and safety services can be provided. The suggested ideas for information booths, displays, demonstrations, and activities are geared to the age and understanding of the child.

Meeting the health and wellness needs of children is notoriously difficult. At this age, getting their attention and maintaining their interest is not the only challenge; now it is also necessary to combat the conflicting messages they receive from the media and peers. It is still important to remember: (1) keep it fun; (2) customize to the age and understanding of the audience.

Goals

To reinforce wellness behaviors via a high-energy, entertaining event

To provide child health screenings and safety services for parents

Target audience

Children age 6–10

Process

- Ideas for partnering:

  YMCA

  PTA

  school science fair, art, or essay contest

- Ideas for incentives:

  school supplies

- Ideas for activities:

  Dunking tank for the "pusher": use a traditional dunk tank, but dress the person being dunked in a criminal-looking outfit and hang a sign above his or her head that says, "Drug Pusher."

Make-your-own healthy snacks: a nutritionist helps children create colorful and tasty snacks. Bring in various shaped cookie cutters to help make the snacks more interesting.

Water balloon toss: create larger-than-life cigarettes from cardboard tubes. Tape a small tin can inside what will be the "lit" end of the cigarette. Place a substance such as incense or other material that smolders easily in the can (you can also use dry ice if it is available). Place the cigarette, smoking end up, in a small children's inflatable pool. After talking to children on the importance of not smoking, give each of them a water balloon and say, "Now let's put out that cigarette for good!" and everyone tosses a balloon at the cigarette.

Pin the food on the pyramid: same concept as "Pin the tail on the donkey." Use cutout shapes of food. The blindfolded child tries to pin the food in the correct quadrant of an empty food pyramid; after each pinning the entire group decides whether the food is in the right place.

Say "No": work with children to practice refusal skills for drugs and inappropriate touch.

Fingerprinting, videotaping.

Challenge course: kids run around a track stopping at fitness stations, where an adult gives them an exercise to perform (jumping jacks, jump rope, push-ups, etc.). Coordinate with a fitness specialist on the number of repetitions appropriate to different age groups.

- Ideas for presentations and demonstrations:

  good habits for athletic success, demonstrated and discussed by athletes

  police/fire department/ambulance service/med-flight teams show children the inside of police car/fire truck/ambulance/helicopter

  "Stop-Drop-Roll" technique for putting out a fire on someone, explained and demonstrated by firefighter

  police dog demonstration

  introduction to medical equipment that a child might see in an office or hospital

  "Being Safe When You Are Home Alone" program for latchkey kids

  first aid and other safety programs for kids

  bicycle, skate, skateboard, and/or helmet safety

- Suggested screenings:
  cholesterol (based on family history)
  immunizations
  blood pressure
  sickle-cell anemia (children of African and Mediterranean heritage)
  dental
  TB
  HIV (for high-risk groups)
  hearing
  respiratory
  scoliosis
  posture
  visual acuity
  learning levels
  speech
  anemia
  lead

Cross-Reference: Chapter 17, Quick Tips; Chapter 20, Preschool Fairs; Chapter 43, Quick Tips; Chapter 48, Circulation Game

22 Preteen/Teen Fairs

A "cooler" version of the elementary school fair targets preteens and teenagers. Teen involvement in putting on the fair is integral. Health screenings, parenting topics, and safety services can be provided. Information booths, displays, demonstrations, and activities are designed to provide objective nonjudgmental information.

Meeting the health and wellness needs of this age group is especially challenging. Negative media messages, peer pressure, natural rebelliousness, and a sense of invulnerability all combine to make getting this group's attention difficult. But it is not impossible, if the messages are presented by people they respect and within their frame of reference.

Goals

To strengthen children's resistance to negative outside messages and pressures

To reinforce positive health messages

To demonstrate healthy role modeling

To offer age-appropriate health screenings

Target audience

Children age 11–18

Process

- Ideas for partnering:

  PTA

  church groups

  YMCA

  youth groups

- Ideas for activities:

  Challenge course: Kids run around a track stopping at fitness stations. A teen or young adult instructs them on an exercise to perform (jumping jacks, jump rope, push-ups, etc.). Coordinate with a fitness specialist on the number of repetitions appropriate to different age groups.

Role playing: Group discusses relevant issues facing teens and the decisions they must make. Then teens role play scenarios given them by the facilitator. After each scenario is played out, the group discusses other options that could have been chosen. Scenarios include dating relationships, saying "no" to drugs/alcohol/tobacco, encountering someone who is depressed or suicidal, defusing a conflict.

- Ideas for presentations and demonstrations (The more involvement of teenagers in presenting the programs, the better. Panel discussions that include teenagers as well as adult experts are highly effective.):

  water safety;

  first aid;

  CPR;

  sexuality: anatomy and physiology of the reproductive system, process of impregnation (including myths on how not to get pregnant), contraception, importance of a committed relationship; consider passing a box around for attendees to put anonymous questions in to be answered by the presenter;

  teen depression;

  overcoming a sense of isolation;

  dealing with academic stress;

  alcohol and drug abuse: consider a panel discussion with a policeman, rehabilitated user, convicted pusher, and family member of someone who died from an overdose;

  sexual abuse (resulting from dates and family);

  STDS/HIV;

  teen pregnancy (myths and realities): include testimonies from one or more single teenage mothers and a teenage couple who married when the girl became pregnant;

  babysitter safety;

  crisis intervention: how to intervene with a peer;

  preteen/teen theaters: Peer education at its best . . . Form a group of preteens and teens who, through presentations, workshops, and theatrical productions, educate their peers about the dangers of HIV/AIDS, unplanned pregnancies, violence, or other relevant topics. Provide the core information and goals of the programs, then let the kids decide how to present it.

- Suggested screenings:

  immunizations

  blood pressure

  dental

  height/weight

  body composition

  cholesterol (based on family history)

  sickle-cell anemia (children of African or Mediterranean heritage)

  visual acuity

  hearing

  STDS/HIV

  hepatitis

  TB

  anemia

- Ideas for displays:

  "Who Wants to Kiss an Ashtray Mouth?" (Paint a large pair of lips on heavy poster board. Tape a jar filled with old used cigarette butts behind the board. Create a tunnel from the mouth of the jar to the lips with plastic. The hole in the mouth allows the teen to put his or her nose in and sniff.)

  statistics on teenage driving accidents under the influence of alcohol or drugs

  divorce rate among teenage married couples

  autopsy cross-sections of cancerous and emphysemic lungs

  pictures of radical surgeries following oral tobacco use

  police department pictures of bodies found from overdoses

  wrecked car(s) displayed from alcohol-related traffic accidents

  nutrition and fitness regimen for training athletes

  list of side effects from anabolic steroids

  statistics on income versus education levels

David Letterman-type poster with "Ten Reasons Why . . . " on any health related topic: why you should eat right, not smoke, wait before having sex, etc. Make some of the answers straightforward, but try to add humor as well.

- Ideas for information/awareness booths:

  local youth programs

  college recruiters

  Alcoholics Anonymous

  Narcotics Anonymous

  representatives from different civilian and military career fields, discussing their professions and counseling youth on scholastic and experiential requirements

  youth support groups

  representatives from a crisis intervention center specializing in youth issues

Cross-Reference: Chapter 17, Quick Tips; Chapter 43, Quick Tips

23 Senior Fairs

A health fair targeting the common needs and interests of aging populations is offered in a supportive and social setting. Customized health screenings, information booths, displays, demonstrations, and special-interest lectures are offered with a focus on maintaining independence and quality of life.

Not only is America aging, but we are living longer and staying active well into our autumn years. As a result the health and wellness needs of this population are changing rapidly. It is important to make senior health fairs a dynamic and positive event.

Goals

To provide screening and information services to aging populations who are not reached adequately by traditional health and wellness programming

To gather metrics concerning future health and wellness needs of this audience

Target audience

Aging populations selected by identified common needs and demographics

Process

- Make sure the entire fair is fully accessible to people with physical limitations.
- Have plenty of places for people to sit and rest.
- Include door-to-door transportation (a nominal fee is okay).
- Ideas for partnering:

  retirement/assisted living facilities

  church groups

  senior centers

  antique fairs, flea markets, arts and crafts fairs
- Ideas for activities:

  eyeglasses repair;

denture checks and minor repairs;

healthy-heart bake sale/cake walk;

games: card games, backgammon, bingo, pool/billiards;

a dance after the health fair;

medication analysis: attendees bring "everything" from their medicine cabinet so that health care professionals can determine any potential problems with drug interactions, overmedicating, etc.;

videos on relevant health topics: post a schedule of when each topic will be shown;

storytelling: set aside a room where a facilitator puts forth topics and encourages participants to tell stories of their experiences related to that topic. Unless there is a valid therapeutic reason to encourage topics that may be depressing, attempt to keep the subjects positive. Topic suggestions include dating, most memorable event revolving around a child or grandchild, ways we entertained ourselves prior to television, vacations, life during the depression, traveling overseas, positive experiences serving in the military (peacetime and war). Another idea is to ask volunteers to "spin the biggest yarn." The audience votes on who told the biggest whopper, and the winner gets a prize.

exercise equipment, with fitness specialists to explain how it works and the benefits; allow attendees to try out the equipment.

- Ideas for presentations and demonstrations:

  adult caregiver issues

  gardening demonstrations

  burglar-proofing your home

  demonstration of simple self-defense techniques

  exercise demonstrations geared toward older populations: strength training; chair exercises; discussions of walking programs; films of aquatic aerobics

  cooking demonstrations for men

  how to interest a "stay-at-home" spouse in outside activities

  financial wellness

- Ideas for screening:

  gout and renal-function checks

blood pressure

blood glucose

potassium

lipid profile

dental

foot checks and nail trimming

skin cancer

Pap smears

breast exams and mammograms

colorectal cancer

vision: acuity, glaucoma, cataracts

hearing

osteoporosis

prostate

flu and pneumonia immunization

- Ideas for information/awareness booths:

legal advice including living wills, estate planning, durable power of attorney for health care, establishing conservatorship/guardianship

nonprofit and self-help organizations such as AARP, Alzheimer's Association, American Heart Association, National Council on Aging, Meals-on-Wheels, etc.

financial counselors

long-term care insurance

emergency response system

professional skilled-home-care organizations

adult day-care facilities

senior centers

retirement facilities

assisted-living facilities

veterans' organizations

representatives from Medicare and the Social Security Administration

"Footprinters"—retired police

- Ideas for displays:

  home security systems

  home water purification systems

  personal emergency response system (transmitter generally worn around the neck or on the wrist, which places a call for help to the nearest emergency response system)

  information on mail order pharmacies

  recommended books

  self-care brochures on common problems found in aging populations: Alzheimer's disease, arthritis, bunions/hammertoes, cataracts, constipation, glaucoma, gout, hair loss, hearing changes, heart and circulatory problems, leg pain, menopause, osteoporosis, prostate problems, skin changes, weakness/fatigue

  laws governing age discrimination

Cross-Reference: Chapter 17, Quick Tips; Chapter 49, Stages of Life; Chapter 50, Independence and Safety; Chapter 51, Staying Connected; Section 8, Resources

24 Parenting Fairs

A health fair focusing on parenting issues provide services, customized health screenings, information booths, displays, demonstrations, and lectures of specific interest. Fair organizers are reminded to consider the unique parenting needs of men as well as women.

The challenges of child rearing are becoming more and more complex, even frightening. Often, parents and other full-time caregivers are unaware of the many services available to them. A community effort to address issues facing parents today will help stabilize the family unit and ultimately increase the chance of children growing into healthy, productive adults.

Goals

To provide parenting information to assist parents in improving parenting skills

To assist parents in need by providing access to community support services

Target audience

Single and married parents as well as full-time, nonparental caregivers

Process

- Provide child care. Consider offering a children's fair in conjunction with the parenting fair. If children are present in some capacity, offer free diapers and a changing area for infants.
- Ideas for partnering:

  PTA

  public health department

  church groups

  social services
- Ideas for activities:

  Children's movies and cartoons: adult volunteers supervise so parents can leave their children while attending the fair.

Parent-child races: usually categorized by mother-daughter or father-son and by age range of the children (other categories could certainly be considered).

Immunization record review: parents bring children's records; health care providers make appropriate recommendations.

Discussion of parent/child confrontations (premarital sex, drugs, smoking, announcing a divorce, dropping out from school, etc.): role-playing scenarios are played out by participants, followed by discussion on other options for dealing with the situation.

- Ideas for presentations and demonstrations:

  helping your child(ren) deal with a divorce, from the perspective of the custodial parent and the noncustodial parent

  Step-parenting/blending families

  discipline techniques

  how to promote self-esteem

  pediatric CPR

  growth and development programs for each pediatric age range

  what to look for: the ingredients of quality child care

  how to spot warning signs of illness, what home treatments to use, and when to call a doctor

  childproofing the home

  helping children deal with death (parents, siblings, friends, relatives)

  building a healthy child: what to do before you get pregnant

  health in childbirth: antenatal and postnatal care

- Ideas for information/awareness booths:

  Big Brother, Big Sister, and mentoring associations

  Women, Infants, and Children's Program (WIC)

  Aid to Families with Dependent Children

  information on food stamps

  parent action and support groups such as Mothers/Dads Against Drunk Driving; Toughlove International; Promise Keepers; Dad's Rights to Parenting

- Ideas for displays:

  importance of reading to children at an early age

  recommended parenting books (consider making them available for purchase)

  names, numbers, and descriptions of family-oriented agencies and toll-free hotlines

Cross-Reference: Chapter 17, Quick Tips; Chapter 20, Preschool Fairs; Chapter 21, Elementary School Fairs; Chapter 22, Preteen/Teen Fairs; Section 8, Resources

25 Men's/Women's Fairs

A health fair targeting gender-specific issues and health needs offers customized health screenings, information booths, displays, demonstrations, and lectures of specific interest.

While all health fairs obviously deal with relevant men and women's health topics, in some situations the complexities of gender-related issues warrant a health fair that focuses on perspectives unique to each sex.

Goals

To provide meaningful services and in-depth information on gender-related issues to a large audience

To gather metrics concerning future health and wellness needs of adult audiences

Target audience

Adults in their 20s through 40s selected by identified common needs and demographics

Process

- Ideas for screening/assessments:

  general: health-risk appraisal and screenings appropriate to either sex

  men: prostate exam/prostate specific antigen, testicular exam, scalp assessment for hair loss

  women: breast exam and mammogram, osteoporosis, anemia, Pap smear
- Ideas for counseling:

  feedback on health-risk appraisal and screenings

  career counseling

  determination of appropriate referral agencies
- Ideas for demonstrations:

  breast self-exam

testicular self-exam

self-defense: general and focusing on women

makeup demonstrations

pregnancy massage

- Ideas for presentations:

  Men

  - dealing with divorce
  - becoming a stepdad
  - emotional health: expressing feelings, aggression, anger management, and competitiveness
  - finding a healthy balance between work, family, and self; the importance of spiritual integration
  - financial program
  - men's cooking class
  - dating in the 90's: a man's perspective
  - sexuality/sexual dysfunction
  - building a healthy relationship with a woman
  - the changing face of workplace relationships: what is harassment, what isn't
  - dress for success

  Women

  - preconception: building a healthy baby
  - stages of pregnancy and delivery
  - dealing with divorce
  - becoming a stepmom
  - sexuality/sexual dysfunction
  - dating in the 90's: a woman's perspective
  - building a healthy relationship with a man
  - "Super Mom" is a myth: balancing home and work
  - pros and cons of hormone replacement therapy

domestic violence and abuse

self-esteem issues

assertiveness

health for women over 50

dealing with menopause

preventing osteoporosis

dealing with stress incontinence

dress for success

basic auto repair/vehicle maintenance

- Ideas for information and awareness booths:

  health care providers/clinics specializing in men's or women's physical and emotional health issues

  counseling services

  nonprofit and community support agencies dealing with some aspect of men's or women's health issues

  social service agencies

  agencies to find "deadbeat" moms/dads

  job placement services

  dating services

- Ideas for displays:

  men's/women's health information

  information on husband abuse and wife abuse

  summaries of laws dealing with gender discrimination, sexual harassment, men's rights in child custody hearings

Cross-Reference: Chapter 17, Quick Tips; Chapter 24, Parenting Fairs; Chapter 26, Focused Health Fairs; Section 8, Resources

26 Focused Health Fairs

These fairs target a specific category or component of health rather than all areas. Topic-related screenings, information booths, displays, demonstrations, and lectures are provided with a depth that would be difficult in more broad-based fairs. The focus remains on how to achieve optimum health in the targeted area.

In every wellness category, many factors affect achieving optimal health. These factors include complex combinations of cultural issues, life experiences, stresses, and work and home environments. By focusing on only one aspect of health, organizers can provide services addressing the issues in enough detail to make the information useful to the majority of attendees.

Goals

To provide meaningful services and in-depth information on a broad category of wellness to a large audience

To gather metrics concerning future health and wellness needs

Target audience

All types, determined by needs assessment prior to health fair

Process

- General principles: regardless of the topic, focused health fairs should be built around these factors:

  assessments of levels of health in the highlighted category (there are many topic-specific assessments available, which provide detailed feedback on areas that need to be addressed; these assessments may be written, verbal, or physical)

  counseling to discuss the findings of any assessments done, as well as answer specific questions presented by the participants

  demonstrations of equipment and/or techniques that can help a person achieve optimal health in the highlighted category

presentations on topics that can be covered adequately in thirty to sixty minutes

information booths of organizations or vendors with products or services relating to the topic

displays of specific information, products, or programs

- Fitness fairs

Ideas for assessments:

percent body fat/weight

strength and flexibility: grip tests, bend and stretch tests, weight lifting, etc.

aerobic capacity via a submaximal stress test

ergonomic assessment of muscle groups used in work environment

overall exercise habits via written or verbal screening

Ideas for counseling:

aerobic program recommendations, including: type of exercise, stages of progression, how to monitor progress, and precautions

strength and flexibility recommendations, ideally with equipment available for demonstration purposes

job specific strength and flexibility recommendations to address unique ergonomic needs

Ideas for demonstrations:

weight training

stretching exercises

aerobic exercise and weight equipment

variety of group exercise programs, including exercise programs for special needs (arthritis, sitting aerobics for people with physical disabilities, children's exercises)

sports massage (include self-help strategies)

proper body mechanics and use of work-related equipment

Ideas for presentations:

discussion of fitness supplements and anabolic steroids

nutrition for the athlete

- sports injuries: how to prevent them and how to treat them
- role of fitness in controlling specific diseases (diabetes, heart disease, arthritis, etc.)
- special programs for physical disabilities
- today's at-risk children: encouraging fitness in sedentary children

Ideas for information and awareness booths:

- personal trainers
- YMCA
- Special Olympics
- martial arts schools
- ergonomic consulting services
- fitness equipment companies

Ideas for displays:

- recommended fitness books
- ergonomic office equipment
- safety equipment
- exercise equipment (all kinds)
- nutrition supplements for peak performance

- Nutrition fairs

Ideas for assessments:

- nutrition analysis
- percent body fat/weight

Ideas for counseling (exercise discretion when using counselors with a commercial weight-loss program affiliation):

- weight management
- therapeutic diets: diabetes, hypoglycemic, low fat

Ideas for demonstrations:

- low-fat cooking
- juicing

preparing healthy desserts and snacks

seasoning options to salt and fat

Ideas for presentations:

basic nutrition/the new Food Pyramid

nutrition needs for the stages of life: pregnancy, childhood, adulthood, aging

eating out and eating right

cooking for one

label reading

grocery store photo tour

vitamins and other nutrition supplements

eating disorders

Ideas for information booths:

representatives from weight-loss programs

representatives from local health food stores

Ideas for displays:

healthy food items (preferably with samples for tasting)

healthy-heart menus from local restaurants

fat/sugar content of unhealthy foods

recommended books on: nutrition, weight management, therapeutic diets

posters with specific nutrition tips, such as getting your child to eat the right foods, choosing foods/liquids for adults/kids when they are sick, getting more calcium in your diet when you don't drink milk, getting more iron in your diet without supplements, helping adults with no appetite get adequate nutrition

- Emotional health fairs

Ideas for assessments:

stress levels

relationships

Ideas for counseling:

focus on referring participants to appropriate support agencies

Ideas for demonstrations:

- biofeedback
- meditation
- yoga
- massage (include self-help strategies)

Ideas for presentations:

- humorist who focuses on therapeutic value of laughter and strategies for bringing humor into the workplace
- developing relaxation skills
- controling your anger
- identifying emotional problems in adults and children, including signs of suicidal thoughts
- spiritual health: strategies for achieving self-awareness, values definition, your purpose for being, the religions/belief systems of the world
- grief and loss programs: death and dying; widow(er)hood; loss of a child, parent; personal health; supporting someone who is dying or grieving
- developing healthy relationships: family, work, social, communication skills
- While many of the programs listed in this section, can be categorized as stressor programs; be sure to consider the following:
  - Work: environmental (noise, lighting, physical demands), management style, shift work
  - Financial health starts with one's attitudes about money, but also includes: retirement, debt management, college funding, budgeting
  - Performance stress: academic, work, family expectations
- mental illness: what is it?
- Pros and cons of mood-altering prescription and over-the-counter drugs

Ideas for information booths:

- crisis centers/hot lines
- religious organizations
- nonprofit emotional health support groups
- financial counselors/planners

- Drug, alcohol, and tobacco awareness fairs

  Ideas for assessments/counseling:

    What is in your medicine cabinet? People bring in all medications, including vitamins and over-the-counter drugs. Look for expired medications and possible interactions, counsel on when and how medications can be taken together (for instance, don't take a calcium supplement at the same time as an iron supplement);

    readiness-to-quit smoking assessment, with follow-up counseling on how to go about it;

    alcohol-use assessment.

  Ideas for demonstrations:

    effects of alcohol on reaction time

    drug-sniffing dog demonstration from police department

    burning of "fake" marijuana so parents/educators know what it smells like

  Ideas for presentations:

    alcohol: is there a problem?

    street drugs: what is out there, what do they do?

    over-the-counter drugs: what is being abused?

    diet and nutrition supplements: pros and cons

    anabolic steroids

    objective information on herbal and homeopathic medications

    oral tobacco: tips for quitting

    smoking: tips for quitting

    making your workplace tobacco/drug free

  Ideas for information booths:

    community drug prevention organizations

    nonprofit support organizations such as Mothers Against Drunk Driving, Alcoholics Anonymous, Narcotics Anonymous

  Ideas for displays:

    autopsy cross-sections of emphysemic or cancerous lungs

oversize display of a mouth with various lesions and problems resulting from oral tobacco use

crime scene pictures of overdose victims

displays of street drugs (so parents can see what they look like)

information on tobacco-cessation aids

statistics related to drug use in the workplace

Cross-Reference: Chapter 17, Quick Tips, Chapter 36, Quick Tips (Grocery store photo tours); Chapter 38, Visual Illustrations of Food Content; Section 8, Resources

Fitness Programming

Generate some good-natured interdepartmental rivalry with this event. It does require a little coordination and staff assistance, but is well worth the effort and does not have to be costly. Besides a variety of traditional fitness activities, include team building and problem solving into the events and become a sure winner with any management interested in improving morale and productivity.

27 Quick Tips

While you're designing and implementing a major fitness program, introduce fitness concepts with these quick tips. Show customers that fitness can be part of everyday life.

- **Fitness and staff meetings**

Who says staff meetings must be held in a conference room? If audiovisual support is not required, get the chairpersons to take meetings outside. While there is a team-building component to attendees going as a group to meeting locations, any physical activity such as walking, running, rollerblading, or biking carries definite benefits. Meeting sites can be anywhere that is relatively quiet (a park, picnic area, fitness trail, etc.). Ideal times for such meetings are immediately before or after lunch or at the end of the day. If membership in such meetings is ten or less, try a walk-and-talk meeting. Use a portable tape recorder to keep a record of the meeting. Provide a transcript to participants later.

- **Exercise-tape lending library**

Music or other forms of auditory entertainment helps pass exercise time for many people. Compile a library of audiocassettes. Walkers and other exercisers check out the tapes, as well as portable cassette players with headphones if they do not have their own. Code musical audiocassettes as slow, medium, and fast-paced for the exerciser wishing to use the tempo to maintain a set workout pace. (Of course, this recommendation assumes outdoor exercising does not occur on busy roads where hearing should not be impaired.) Other ideas: include culturally diverse music and self-improvement tapes in your checkout library.

- **In-house walking track**

Do you have employees who cannot leave the building during their work shift? Establish a walking course in the building. Measure out and post the number of circuits necessary to equal one mile on this "track." Establish a set direction for all exercisers, to minimize hallway congestion. Change the direction of the course weekly to minimize ankle strain. Establish set hours for exercise. Coordinate with housekeeping. Exercise rules should include a requirement that walkers must stay to the right, housekeeping keeps all equipment to the left, and nonexercisers walk to the left during exercise hours.

■ Worksite exercise areas

Often worksite fitness centers are underutilized because employees find it hard to get away from their immediate work area. Set up a mobile fitness center—you take equipment to the work area, either on permanent loan or for certain hours or days of the week. Establish a rotating schedule for multiple worksites. Some type of accountability may be necessary to ensure the security of equipment. Put punching bags in employee restrooms. Punching bags are cheap, convenient, and don't take up a lot of room. Just a few minutes of punching the bag carries a significant aerobic benefit, helps wake up the "punchy" employee who has been sitting at a desk, and can be a terrific tension reliever during a stressful day.

■ "Beat the boss" program

Find one or more senior managers who are relatively competitive in some type of aerobic exercise. Ask the managers to exert maximum effort at their exercise of choice under controlled conditions. Record their best time. Then challenge the rest of the organization to "beat the boss." Offer a prize for every employee who can beat the official time set by the manager. This can be an ongoing challenge, spanning an entire year, or a lead-in to a one-time group fitness activity.

■ Fitness lottery

Find one or more respected senior managers who are willing to exercise with groups of employees on a periodic basis. This group exercise can be weekly, monthly, quarterly, or whatever commitment you can get from the managers, but it must be a firm commitment. The managers do not have to be excellent athletes, but should recognize the importance their presence brings to motivating employee participation. Promote the activity as a prestigious event. Limit the size of each exercise group by drawing names for the privilege of exercising with these managers.

■ Cardiovascular room videos

If cardiovascular rooms offer televisions for exercisers to watch during workouts, connect a VCR and offer wellness tapes instead of the usual television shows. Screen the tapes to ensure they are high quality and not too lengthy. There may be a little complaining at first, but once the tapes become part of their fitness routine most exercisers will watch them and appreciate access to the information.

■ Encouraging use of stairwells

What can you do to encourage use of building stairwells over elevators? Make them more interesting. Do you sponsor art contests? Post the entries in the stairwells. Put up bulletin boards, announcements, or cartoons. Start stair-climbing competitions. How do the stairwells look? Correct any problems with lighting or a dingy appearance. Hang seasonal decorations. Coordinate plans with the necessary safety officials.

- **"Secrets of the super models"**

Search for a fitness trainer who works with models or beauty contestants. Ask him or her to speak on training protocols and other advice given to clients. It is certainly a good idea to screen these protocols; but assuming they are an appropriate balance of aerobic conditioning, toning, and nutrition, a program promoted as revealing the "secrets of the super models" is a surefire draw for women of virtually any age. A similar men's program can be offered by a fitness trainer to competitive bodybuilders.

- **Customized aerobic music**

Not everyone enjoys the same type of music. This may be particularly true if you are targeting a certain ethnic group or age range. If it is not feasible to offer each target audience's preferred music all the time, select certain days each week or month. Once target-audience members start participating on their "special days," they will be more inclined to attend all the time. Promote the aerobics classes with special upbeat titles such as "Reggae Aerobics Night" or "Jazzercizing to the 'Big Band Sound.'" For a change of pace, offer seasonal or holiday music. Consider classes set to the soundtracks from favorite movies.

- **Exercise videos**

Build your own library of exercise videos for individual checkout, in-house cable, or organized group activities. Film a video of senior managers exercising. This can be a really popular video with employees, and it demonstrates that management values fitness and that they are willing to poke a little fun at themselves. Sponsor an interdepartmental competition to produce the best exercise video. Or assign a different type of exercise to be developed by a department or volunteer group (e.g., bodybuilding, jazzercise, boxing, aerobics, tai chi). Develop work-hardening exercise videos that focus on movements or muscle groups required for performing a job-related task.

- **Entertainment and fun runs**

Turn a fun run into a unique event by sponsoring entertainment along the route. Provide live or taped music, magicians, jugglers, clowns, mimes, cheerleaders, short skits, or anything else your imagination can dream up and resources can support. Economical sources for the entertainment can include scout troops, the chamber of commerce, local theater groups, entertainers looking for exposure, civic organizations, United Way agencies, and schools. Encourage participation by sponsoring a contest to award the best entertainment.

- **Weight room hours**

Novice bodybuilders, people who lack confidence in their appearance and/or ability, and seniors are frequently intimidated when working in weight rooms with typical young buffed-up athletes. Consequently, they stay away altogether. Monitor utilization trends in the weight room. Select hours where usage is lowest and limit use of the room to one or more of these groups. If possible, have coaches with a similar background to this audience present during these special hours.

- **Choosing aerobic instructors**

Select your aerobic instructors according to the specific target audience. Senior citizens or the significantly overweight find it difficult to relate to the perky, skinny-as-a-rail aerobic instructor. Ethnicity or gender may be an issue. If it is not feasible to hire a number of diverse instructors, consider a certification program, where laypeople are trained and monitored by a qualified instructor to lead classes in a routine developed by the instructor for their target audience.

- **Self- and assisted-massage programs**

Sports massage has gained significant popularity among athletes. There are many simple self- and assisted-massage techniques that can be taught to laypeople to enhance performance, minimize injury, and speed recovery when an injury occurs. Besides ensuring that the massage therapist specializes in the types of therapeutic massage you need, screen for licenses or certificates, references, school graduated from, and extra credit hours accrued. Just as important, how well can they impart information? A good massage therapist is not necessarily a good speaker. Self- and assisted-massage programs are equally effective as part of a back, neck, or headache program and as a tool to combat the effects of stress.

28 Costumed Fun Run

Exercise time becomes a pleasure when you are having a good time. Throw elements of creativity, fashion, and fun into your next fun run. Consider thematic fun runs, where the running outfits and accessories, as well as running times, are judged. Theme runs can also assume a paradelike atmosphere.

People will offer many reasons for not participating in organized fitness programs. Two common excuses are "It's boring" and "I could never do as well as the more fit participants." Adding elements of fun and opportunities for the less fit to be recognized in a competitive environment help attract this large audience segment. Additionally, people with similar interests are attracted to events that offer opportunities to interact socially.

Goals

To increase participation in fitness events

To demonstrate that fitness can be enjoyable

To stimulate participant interaction and bonding

Target audience

All types

Process

- Develop a fun-run calendar based on themes to which the target audiences can relate.
- Fun-run promotion should include this information:

  definition of fun-run theme

  ideas for costumes/accessories (including safety considerations)

  judging criteria and awards for winners
- Awards for participation in costume/theme fun runs can be based on any combination of the following criteria:

  best costumes/accessories

compliance with fun-run theme

highest percentage of departments/organizations represented

best running/walking times

overall

If costumes or accessories would reasonably slow down a good runner, differentiate between best running/walking times for participants who are not in costume and those who are.

- Avoid themes that would necessitate complex costumes or props or present risk of overheating or injury.
- Ideas for themes:

Holidays

Halloween: prize for best costume

Mardi Gras: prize for best costume

Christmas: elves, reindeer, Santa, running teams dressed as each of the twelve days of Christmas

Independence Day: runners carrying flags, sparklers (nighttime runs)

Valentine's Day: runners wearing large valentines with loved one's name on their chests

Seasons

Winter: jingle bell run—small bells laced into running shoes

Dog Days of Summer: hosing stations throughout course to cool off runners

Ides of March: short togas made from sheets, with olive-branch sweatbands

Cultural recognitions

Cinco de Mayo: fiesta-type costumes

Okctoberfest: volkesmarch with German costumes

Hobbies/special interests

Mutt Strut: participants run/walk with their dogs—concept can be expanded to include other pets (some may have to be carried)

Reading: favorite book character

Professional sports (football, basketball, baseball, etc.): team jerseys/colors

Popular entertainment icons

Elvis's birthday: Elvis lookalike runners

Star Trek: runners dress as their favorite alien

Organizational mission

Departmental: T-shirts that differentiate between departments

Medical organization: MASH run

- Where possible, select judges who are from senior management or are well-respected members of the community.
- Vary the frequency of thematic fun runs based on popularity, but once a month is probably a good average. If frequent fun runs are the norm or goal, more traditional fun runs (held throughout the month) will support the thematic runs as target audiences become motivated to perform well.

Variations

- Thematic relay races—Example: Christmas Relay Race

  Relay could be done as a communitywide event or an interdepartmental challenge within a large organization. Teams of eight runners wearing reindeer antlers pull a Santa in his sleigh (lightweight vehicle on wheels). As a community run, this could be done as an event by itself or as part of a parade. Santa is "handed off" to other teams of eight at set intervals until course is completed.

  Runners who wish to run the course but not participate in the relay escort the teams wearing elf costumes.

- Community costume/theme fun runs/walks

  Have a longer course, preferably winding through town. Scenic areas are a plus. Consider entertainment along route. If awards are to be offered, registration may be necessary, and nonregistered participants can join anywhere along course, but are not eligible for awards.

Cross-Reference: Chapter 1, Quick Tips (Incentives); Chapter 27, Quick Tips (Entertainment and Fun Runs); Chapter 29, Scavenger Hunt Fun Runs; Chapter 30, Murder Mystery Fun Runs

29 Scavenger Hunt Fun Run

Remember the old scavenger hunts of your youth? This fun run incorporates the basic rules of an old favorite party game into a group activity that encourages socializing, problem solving, and fitness in one popular event. Great as an organizational or community event.

Goals

To increase participation in fitness events

To demonstrate that fitness can be enjoyable

To stimulate participant interaction and bonding

Target audience

Adults and older teenagers

Process

- Scavenger hunt fun runs provide opportunities for participants to meet people outside their normal sphere of friends and acquaintances.

  As an organizational event, it is especially effective for large corporations with closely located buildings. Employees become familiar with other departments.

  As a community event, neighbors meet neighbors.

  Commercial businesses can use the opportunity to promote their company to potential customers.
- Identify homes, offices, or businesses that agree to allow scavengers to visit.
- Provide them with a sign to place on their doors, indicating their participation as a scavenger hunt site.
- Develop a list of small, lightweight items that could reasonably be available in these sites and not need to be returned.

  Examples of office handouts:

  colored paper clips or Post-it notes

  letterhead paper

interoffice mailer

empty water/juice container or healthy snack wrapper

health promotion brochure or program calendar

Examples of commercial business handouts:

small promotional items with a business logo/address, such as pencils, refrigerator magnets, balloons

carry out menu

Examples of home handouts:

healthy-heart recipe

old fitness accessories: sweatband, running sock, running-shoe lace, fitness event T-shirt

a piece of a healthy snack: dried fruit, pretzel, carrot stick

empty nicotine-replacement therapy wrapper/container (patch, gum, etc.)

- Allocate points to each item on the scavenger hunt list. Points can be all the same or weighted based on anticipated difficulty in finding.
- Instruct runners/walkers to

  wear a fanny pack or lightweight knapsack on day of race;

  approach only offices, businesses, or homes with the appropriate sign indicating their participation in the scavenger hunt;

  take only one item per scavenger site (inform participating sites of this rule).
- To determine the winners, score runners and walkers not participating in the hunt separately from scavengers—winners are determined by their running/walking times.

  Winners of the scavenger hunt are determined by subtracting the appropriate number of points for each item gathered from the running/walking time; lowest score wins. Example:

  Running time: 2 hours (120 minutes)

  Found 10 items: each item is worth 5 points

  Score: 120 minus 50 = 70 points

Cross-Reference: Chapter 28, Costumed Fun Run; Chapter 30, Murder Mystery Fun Run

30 Murder Mystery Fun Run

Tap into the universal love of a good murder mystery. Along the fun-run course participants gain clues to a murder; then they solve the crime at the end of the event. Even couch potatoes can have a role in this entertaining fitness activity.

This event will capture the interest of people who place reading first on their list of hobbies.

Goals

To increase participation in fitness events

To demonstrate that fitness can be enjoyable

To stimulate participant interaction and bonding

Target audience

Assuming a one-third to one-half participation rate, this activity is ideally suited for moderate-sized organizations or groups of about 100 adults or teenagers

Process

- This is an ideal activity held in conjunction with an organizational picnic or similar social event.
- Prior to the fun-run, form a small planning group to "plot" the murder. Members should have a good background knowledge of the target audience:

  hobbies/special interests

  places they have visited or lived in the past

  connections (past or present) with other members of the target audience

  current and past jobs
- Based on this information, choose five or six people to be "suspects" in the murder and one to be a "victim." One of the suspects will actually become the "murderer" of the victim.

  Create reasons why all the suspects should want to "kill" the victim by working true background information into a story line. Be as outrageous as you want with reality. Examples:

Turn a hobby into a cover for a smuggling operation. The suspect could be smuggling diamonds over international borders, using the hobby as a front. The victim has discovered this secret and wants in on the action.

The suspect and victim knew each other since childhood and share some dark secret. The victim is wracked with guilt and wants to come forward with the truth. The suspect wants to keep that from happening at any cost.

Find some way to place blame on the victim for some well-known (or made-up) office problem that has created problems for the suspect.

All the suspects should have good reasons to kill the victim, but choose one to actually be the murderer.

Try to choose suspects and a victim who have a sense of humor and are naturally outgoing. You want people who will play their parts with zeal.

- Once the story line has been developed, contact the people you have chosen to be in the murder mystery and ensure their cooperation. Swear all participants to secrecy. No one is to reveal their secrets ahead of time, and definitely not the identity of the murderer.

  It's always a good idea to have one or two more suspects than you really need. Invariably, something comes up and one of the players has to bow out at the last minute.

- Provide each suspect with a description of his/her reason for killing the victim and a different piece of information each suspect can use to divert attention to another suspect. For instance, if the victim is to be shot, one suspect can mention that he or she observed another suspect target practicing a few days earlier.

  The suspects should know nothing about their fellow suspects' reasons for wanting to kill the victim beyond the one diversionary clue each is given.

- The murderer is given the necessary additional information on when, where, and how the murder is to happen.
- Approximately ten volunteer support personnel can effectively work with thirty to forty runners and walkers. Larger crowds can be accommodated but represent a more complex logistical challenge.

Besides the suspects, murderer, and victim, nonrunning participants are needed to fill these positions:

group facilitator (Inspector Clueseau) to help solve the murder

starter and timer at finish line

recorder of finishing times

- Prior to the run, Inspector Clueseau informs the runners/walkers that there are suspicious goings-on within the organization and that he or she fears "something awful will happen" if they can't get to the bottom of the problem soon. The inspector needs their help. If runners encounter people acting suspiciously along the course, they should engage them in conversation and try to determine their part in this mystery.
- Position each suspect at a set point along the running course. The first point should be far enough into the run to allow participants to spread out.

  As small groups of runners come up to a suspect, he or she should melodramatically act out his or her frustration, anger, sorrow, or whatever is needed for the role.

  Suspects should make the runners probe a little for their secret, but help guide their inquiries. For instance, if the secret involves something that happened in the suspect's childhood, he or she can say, "It's just not fair! One mistake years ago shouldn't be held against me now."

  To keep the runners moving along the course, the secret should be released within one or two minutes of questioning.
- It's a good idea to test the course ahead of time to determine how long it would take an average fast walker to get to each suspect's position (and allow for about two minutes for talking at each point). Based on that information, instruct the suspects to head for the finish line at the times you have determined the last of the average walkers will have gone through. A few stragglers may still be on the course, but you have to draw the line somewhere.
- While waiting for the runners/walkers to come in from the course, plan activities to keep participants occupied, such as awards for best running/walking times, food, beverages.

  Inspector Clueseau can encourage participants to share the clues they learned along the course.

The (soon-to-be) victim has a role here in responding to questions about clues that obviously relate to him or her. The victim can act as coldhearted and dastardly as he or she wants. The victim should answer questions accurately, but not make it too easy for the audience. Make them probe for answers.

Don't let the audience totally focus on the victim. Encourage cross-talk among them.

- After the bulk of the runners are in, it is time for the murder. This can happen one of two ways:

  play out the murder in front of the audience;

  someone finds the victim already dead.

- Inspector Clueseau gathers the participants around the body, looks for clues, and begins asking questions. Encourage the audience to share their ideas and ask questions of the suspects. Suspects can use their diversionary clues to avoid interrogation. Don't let the audience totally focus on the suspects. Encourage cross-talk among them.

  If the organization has adopted Total Quality Management (TQM) techniques, attempt to use TQM problem-solving clues in solving the crime (management will love this!).

- A winner is declared when someone correctly guesses who did it and why.
- If the crime can't be solved within an hour, there is no winner.

  Inspector Clueseau instructs each suspect to state his or her reasons for "hating" the victim, but they swear they didn't commit the crime. The "murderer" is the last to state his or her reasons and confesses to the crime.

- Note: A tremendous side-benefit to this activity is the team-building spirit it can generate among the participants. The opportunity to role-play allows participants to bring down natural barriers as they socialize. Participants get to know each other better as they dig for the clues buried in real information about the players' lives.

Variations

Allowing the suspects to drop clues one or two days before the fun run is an excellent marketing strategy and builds interest in the activity. Frequently, participants you would normally not see at fitness events will participate out of curiosity. A word of caution: if you choose this variation, there may be a slight decline in productivity during those days, because people will be talking to each other more to learn clues.

A number of commercially made role-playing murder games are on the market. Such games could easily be incorporated into a fun run and would eliminate some of the logistical work in developing the story line and clues. However, since the plot would not be based on the real lives of participants, some of the personal interaction would be lost.

31 Personal-Best Competition

When trying to improve your level of fitness, the best person to compete against is yourself. This competition does just that, but in a structure that allows for ongoing monitoring, coaching, and incentives.

Often novice runners set unrealistic expectations for themselves by comparing their progress with other, more experienced runners' achievements. Such comparisons cause frustration and disappointment and may ultimately lead to giving up altogether. This program rewards individual progress, provides the motivation and incentive of a competition, but remains achievable for anyone at any fitness level.

Goal

To motivate individuals to develop and maintain a personal exercise program

Target audience

All types

Process

- The purpose of the personal-best competition is to allow participants to measure and be rewarded for their own progress in achieving personal fitness.
- The course does not need to be long. Relatively short courses, of no more than one to three miles, are less daunting to novice runners. Shorter courses also allow the health promotion staff to manage a number of competitions in one day.
- If competitions are held at set intervals throughout the year (ideally every one to three months), participants have milestones that motivate them to maintain an exercise program.
- Anyone can enter the program at any point in the year during one of the competitions.
- The health promotion department posts a sign-up sheet for competitors prior to the event. Competitors sign up for a running time convenient for them.
- The health promotion department maintains a record on each competitor to

track the date they enter the program, all running times, awards, problems, and counseling/training sessions occurring throughout the year.

- New enrollees are screened for preexisting health problems that may contraindicate running and are counseled on warm-ups, cool-downs, and other safety issues.
- Depending on the number of participants, the competition can be run individually or in small groups. Groups may be more convenient for a small health promotion staff, but allow less personalized counseling time.

  Since they will need more initial counseling, it may be wise to run new enrollees in separate groups from other competitors.

  At every race, remind competitors that they are only trying to beat their own best recorded running time.
- To receive an award initially, runners must beat their baseline running time. In subsequent competitions, runners must beat their best time ever in any of the competitions. All runners who run a "personal best" receive a prize. Ideally, the awards ceremony should be a special event for all competitors, held at the end of the day. First-time runners are establishing a baseline for subsequent competitions and do not receive a prize.
- It should be a local decision as to whether competitors must run in every competition throughout the year in order to stay enrolled in the program. Allowing one competition to be missed in a year is probably appropriate. At some point, the runner should be required to reenroll as a new competitor.

Variation

Although designed as a running competition, the concept can be easily modified to other forms of exercise and to physical disabilities.

Cross-Reference: Chapter 1, Quick Tips (Incentives)

32 Adopt-a-Spud Program

Tap into the knowledge and enthusiasm of the fitness "jocks" in your target audience. Partner them with couch potatoes (who aspire to be more) as a prelude to a fitness event that jointly rewards the finishing time of both partners.

Previously sedentary individuals starting out on a fitness program frequently become frustrated and lose their motivation. Personalized one-on-one counseling and coaching is a strong motivator, but difficult for a limited health-and-wellness staff. Peer support from fitness-oriented individuals can be a valuable adjunct to a structured fitness program.

Goals

To provide a meaningful support system to sedentary audiences

To reinforce healthy fitness concepts in already motivated audiences

Target audience

All types

Process

- Schedule a beginners' fitness program offering the usual spectrum of services, information, and assessments available to the novice athlete.
- The entire program should ideally span a number of client interactions and include the following:

  fitness assessment

  body fat and/or weight measurements

  physical and emotional benefits of fitness

  medical evaluation and clearance as necessary

  protocols for beginning and advancing in an exercise program

  counseling and reevaluation
- Schedule a running and/or race-walking competition six to eight weeks from the beginning of the fitness program.

- Marketing of the competition:

  to the novice runner or walker—promote the competition as a culmination to the beginners' fitness program

  to the experienced athlete—initiate an aggressive promotion campaign outlining the requirements that they must agree to "adopt" someone from the beginners' fitness program and coach them over the ensuing weeks

  The better the prizes, the better the participation and motivation of both the experienced athletes and novices.

- Consider holding a raffle or some other type of special recognition for the volunteer adopters after the race as an added incentive.
- Offer a special coaching class for the "adopters," covering these aspects:

  expectations of the "adopters"

  training protocols for beginners

  nutrition and other related lifestyle issues

  motivation tips

  inappropriate training

  dealing with problems such as frustration, injuries, etc.

- Rules of the race:

  Length of the race should be no more than three to five miles.

  If race-walking is part of the event, it is best to hold the competition on a track where the entire course can be viewed to ensure competitors walk the entire race.

  The race involves teams of two: a novice and an experienced racer.

  Team placement is based on best cumulative times.

33 Climb a Mountain, Swim a Sea, Bike across America

Sponsor a race inside your fitness center—participants never leave the building. This simple, inexpensive contest generates enthusiasm and adds an element of competition to daily aerobic exercise.

Competition is a proven motivator for many people. Even low-profile in-house competitions increase enthusiasm among participants.

Goals

To encourage use of fitness center equipment and/or swimming pool

To increase audience motivation to maintain an ongoing fitness program

Target audience

All types, although most often used in conjunction with a worksite wellness program

Process

- All aerobic equipment used must have automatic monitors to measure the amount of individual usage. Different competitions can be run concurrently for each type of equipment available in the center (stair-steppers, rowing machines, treadmills, stationary bicycles, etc.). Since an increase in usage of the aerobic equipment can be anticipated as the competition progresses, more than one piece of each type of equipment is recommended. A swimming pool can be used for a competition if a lifeguard is on duty to count participant laps.
- Develop a chart that pictorially illustrates the type of race the equipment being used represents. Use a poster-size blowup of a real picture, map, or drawing of some well-known landmark (mountain, cross-country terrain, large lake or ocean).

  Measure off the length or height of the landmark on the chart in feet or mile increments.

Include a place on the chart to show the names of participants as they progress toward the finish line (climbing the mountain, crossing the lake/ocean/country).

Post the chart(s) in a highly visible place in the fitness center or organization.

- These rules of the competition apply to a stair-stepper, but they can be modified for any other type of equipment. Announce the day the competition(s) will begin. Participants must register with the fitness center staff, who will start a record for each contestant. Besides the usual demographic information on each participant, the record will show each visit to the fitness center, which stairstepper is used, the amount of feet climbed in each session, and a cumulative total since the beginning of the competition.
- When a participant comes to the fitness center for each workout session, he or she notifies a staff member. A staff member accompanies the participant to the stairstepper and ensures that the monitor is zeroed out prior to use; at the end of the session, the staff member notes the number of feet/miles climbed on the participant's record. The participant records are kept by the fitness center staff.
- Staff members update the competition chart on an ongoing basis. Each time the participants accrue a required number of feet, their names are moved an appropriate amount up the mountain toward the finish line.
- When a participant reaches the mountaintop, the winner is declared and a new competition starts. Use the same mountain to streamline reproduction costs, although different landmarks help keep the competition fresh and interesting.
- Any award or incentive can be used, but a popular approach for this type of competition is to offer a T-shirt that says, "I Climbed Mount Kilimanjaro" (or whatever).

34 Twelve Bosses before Christmas

Help customers keep off those unwanted pounds over the holiday season, and at the same time, send a highly visible message that management supports health. This twelve-day holiday exercise program is fun and guaranteed to be well attended.

The holiday season between Thanksgiving and Christmas is traditionally one of the most difficult times of the year for people to maintain a fitness program. Yet, because people tend to take in more calories during this time of year, it is especially important that they exercise. Any fitness activity that involves management is bound to improve lackluster attendance.

Goals

To encourage exercise during the holiday season

To demonstrate management's support of the health promotion program

To stimulate management interest in the healthy promotion program

Target audience

Worksite employees

Process

- Enlist the cooperation of at least twelve senior managers from the workplace. To ensure maximum marketing penetration throughout the company, encourage managers who supervise a variety of departments to participate.
- Assign each manager a day leading up to Christmas to lead an exercise activity with company employees. The activities can be any combination of group aerobic exercises ranging from dance aerobics to a fun run to bicycling. Base the decision on the managers' personal exercise preferences and/or the capabilities of the workplace to accommodate different types of exercising.
- If the manager is a novice exerciser but willing to participate, offer to coach him or her in an exercise of interest prior to the assigned day. Another alternative is for the inexperienced manager to colead an aerobic exercise group with a trained instructor.

- Build marketing strategies around the holiday song "The Twelve Days of Christmas." For example,

  "On the first day of Christmas,
  the CEO gave to me . . .
  a one-mile fun run.

  On the second day of Christmas,
  the maintenance department director gave to me . . .
  two jumping jacks in his aerobic class.

  On the third day of Christmas,
  the finance officer gave to me . . .
  three miles biking, etc."

  It is not necessary to confine the exercise to that mentioned in the song, but seek to include it as part of the day's routine.

- Participating managers are expected to promote the entire twelve-day program among their employees.
- Any ideas to add fun and a holiday feeling to the exercise sessions will increase the appeal and draw greater participation as subsequent sessions are held:

  managers wear Santa's hats while they exercise

  participants tie small jingle bells on their exercise shoes

  holiday music plays in the background

35 Fitness Week

Generate some good-natured interdepartmental rivalry with this event. It does require a little coordination and staff assistance, but is well worth the effort and does not have to be costly. Besides a variety of traditional fitness activities, include team building and problem solving into the events and become a sure winner with any management interested in improving morale and productivity.

Initial exposure to new fitness activities should be a positive experience. Group settings where the focus is excitement and a positive social atmosphere accomplish this goal. Exposing people to a variety of fitness and recreational activities increases the chance they will find an activity to enjoy for a lifetime.

Goals

To expose participants to a wide variety of fitness and recreational activities

To involve participants, regardless of fitness levels, in group fitness activities

To enhance problem-solving skills

To build team spirit, cohesiveness, and morale

Target audience

Large organizations with multiple departments; easily modifiable for interorganizational competitions

Process

- This fitness event is meant to span a five-day work week, but could be modified to other lengths. A different event is held each day.

  Winners of each event gain points for their sponsoring department. The department with the most accumulated points at the end of the week is declared the winner.

- For maximum effectiveness, make "Fitness Week" a recurring, major organizational event.

  Tap into natural interdepartmental competitiveness by establishing a "rotating" prize or trophy. The department with the most accumulated points at the end of the week wins the right to hold and proudly display the prize until the next "Fitness Week."

- Each day's event focuses on one or more elements of fitness.

  Aerobic exercise—individual and group competitions:

    race walking

    relay races

    running

    swimming

  Strength/flexibility—individual and group competitions:

    carrying buckets of sand a set number of feet in the shortest period of time

    pulling a sled, car, or other piece of equipment a set number of feet in the shortest period of time

    lifting free weights

  Sports and recreation:

    basketball elimination tournament

    touch football elimination tournament

    "best ball" golf tournament

  Obstacle course—team must cross the course using problem solving and teamwork. Ideas for creating the obstacle course:

    ready-made fitness challenge courses

    children's playground equipment

    hiking trails

  Create a task that must be accomplished through teamwork, problem solving, and a moderate amount of physical exertion. Each team's goal is to accomplish the task within a predetermined maximum time and have the best time of all competing teams.

  Provide the team with some basic resources that may (or may not) be helpful in accomplishing their task (e.g., 2 x 4s, ropes, tape, toolbox, timer).

  Incorporate obstacles to accomplishing the task. Obstacles can be a physical challenge in the course or restrictions on how the team proceeds through the course. Allot penalties in time lost for any infraction of the rules or restrictions.

Possible restrictions:

no talking allowed in part (or all) of the course;

certain areas of the obstacle or course cannot be touched or walked upon, but must still be crossed;

everyone must complete the course and task together;

one team-member is injured (blind, broken leg/arm, etc.).

A referee accompanies each team through the course to

explain the challenge, rules, and course;

act as timer;

enforce time-loss penalties for infractions;

determine whether the task has been successfully accomplished.

- Depending on the type of competition, winning points are awarded for the following achievements:

  the best collective racing times per departmental team

  the placing of departmental teams in sporting events (i.e., first, second, third place equal 30, 20, 10 points)

  the placing of individual departmental competitors (i.e., first, second, third place equal 3, 2, 1 points)

- Team selection

  Define the departments from which teams can be organized.

  Avoid making this event a competition of departmental "jocks." It is important to ensure all employees are equally involved in each event. This can be accomplished in one of two ways:

  random selection of teams and department representatives (employees with the same last number of company identification number, employees with the same first number of social security number, every third person selected from an alphabetical roster, etc.)

  criteria for team composition proportional to the demographics found within the workforce (age groups, genders, weight, management/blue-collar, career field, etc.)

- In order for departments to begin preparing for "Fitness Week," all competitions should be explained well in advance of the event. All members will be encouraged to practice since they may be on a team. Specific team composition should be announced at the last possible moment.

Allow time for necessary work schedule adjustments.

Allow time for a review of health records or physical waivers. Make adjustments to teams as necessary where physical restrictions exist.

- Nonparticipants should certainly be encouraged to watch the events and cheer on their favorite teams. However, if "Fitness Week" is being held during a normal work day, post a schedule of when individuals or teams are expected to be present to allow departments minimal loss of needed workforce. The schedule should show the following:

  when each round is expected to start and which departments are playing (sporting events such as basketball, football, or baseball will usually accommodate only two teams playing at once).

  when and where each team/individual must report to play

  if appropriate, transportation drop-off and pickup times

- At the end of each day's competitions, hold an award ceremony for participants to

  congratulate the day's winning teams and individuals;

  declare the total points won by each department that day;

  update current departmental standings for the week's big award.

Variation

Add an additional element of fun by connecting the fitness events to the work environment or ergonomic challenges:

warehouse employees: box loading

medical personnel: wheelchair races, litter carrying

heavy equipment operators: pulling tractor (with brakes off), disassembling and reassembling a piece of equipment

firefighters: extinguishing a giant smoking cigarette

Nutrition Programming

36 Quick Tips

Give everyone in the company a chance to improve their nutritional knowledge and their eating habits. Many of these quick tips can be implemented at little cost, but can make a big change in healthy eating habits.

- **Healthy-heart potluck/brown-bag lunches**

Coordinate periodic employee potluck or brown-bag lunches by assigning each employee a different healthy-heart food item to bring. Provide guidelines on the dos and don'ts of healthy-heart cooking. If participants are new to the concept of healthy-heart cooking, provide them with recipes to test on each other. Generally, keep food item assignments as simple as possible, although occasional more elaborate meals may be well received. Consider the constraints of worksite eating, for example, refrigerator space, food heating/reheating, and storage.

- **Office working lunches**

Generally, senior executive secretaries are responsible for coordinating working lunches for staff members. Get to know the secretaries and convert them to the joys of healthy eating; then provide them with menus from restaurants that serve healthier food items. Highlight the healthy-heart food selections from the menus for them. The easier you can make their demanding jobs, the better. They will appreciate the help.

- **Office social events**

Contact the coordinators of office picnics and cookouts. Provide them with ideas for healthy-heart options, such as grilled chicken breasts, turkey hot dogs/hamburgers, and vegetable kabobs. Don't insist on all healthy-heart foods; just ask that a choice be available. If you meet resistance, survey employees. Often these surveys reflect that, while employees will eat virtually anything provided, they would choose healthier options if they were available. Review items available in break rooms for snacking. Attempt to integrate such items as bagels and nonfat cream cheese or fruit spreads for morning breaks and air-popped popcorn for later in the day. Offer lower-fat options for special events such as birthdays. Find local bakeries that have low-fat cake and icing options. Offer nonfat ice cream and frozen yogurt.

■ **Vending machines**

Typically, vending machine companies do not stock healthy snacks because they are more costly than the fatty and sugary counterparts. If there is a contractual agreement defining services provided by the vending machine company, seek to have a percentage of healthy-heart items required in the contract. Another strategy is to ask the vending machine operators to slightly raise the cost of the fatty and sugary snacks and make a commensurate lowering of prices for the healthier snacks. It is important to promote this addition of healthier food items in vending machines to employees. Often the more health-conscious employees have stopped looking in the vending machines because they have given up on finding anything that is healthy.

■ **Self-guided grocery store tours**

Map out the location of food item categories in local grocery stores. Develop a grocery store tour script reflecting the physical layout of the food items and unique characteristics of each participating store. Tape the program on an audiocassette, indicating when the listener should stop the tape and where to go in the store before starting the tape again. Enlist the aid of store managers to post small signs or flags to help participants find the next listening point. Most stores will be very happy to cooperate, since the program is an excellent promotional strategy. Reproduce a number of the cassettes for each participating store and purchase an appropriate number of portable cassette players with headphones and small journals for taking notes. The journal can be used to validate participants using the tape if any type of incentive is being offered. The grocery stores may be willing to maintain the journals, tapes, and portable cassette players for check-out within the store, but it is probably more reasonable to maintain the necessary materials in the health promotion office.

■ **Grocery store slide tours**

For various reasons, many people are not willing to spend the time or are not physically able to expend the necessary energy for a walking grocery store tour. By photographing store aisles, food placement, and other aspects of a typical grocery store tour, the health promotion manager can take a 35mm slide tour to the audience. Grocery store slide tours reach larger audiences and allow for customization. For instance, parents may be interested in how to shop for healthy food items for their children, or single adults may be interested in easy-to-fix foods. Program presenters can focus on ethnic foods for diverse audiences or on the needs of high-risk audiences, such as diabetics or cardiac patients. Based on audience needs, the program presenter highlights the areas of interest. Slide tours also allow the program presenter to modify the length to fit time constraints.

- **Cooking shows**

Julia Child, Martha Stewart, Graham Kerr, and others like them have all discovered that people like to watch recipes being prepared. Offer periodic healthy-heart cooking shows in the health promotion department or some other convenient locale, such as a cafeteria. If the organization has an in-house cable system, tape the shows and run them on an ongoing basis. The cooking can be done by a health promotion staff member or by a popular layperson. Another strategy is to have a guest cook from the target audience assist the experienced cook. Each show should provide the recipe of the day. Depending on how often the shows are offered, consider periodically compiling the recipes into a cookbook. The cookbooks can be handed out to anyone or used as incentives, prizes, or fund-raisers.

37 Team-Based Weight-Loss Programs

Build a support system into your weight-loss program. This three-month program partners teams with similar weight-loss goals and should be offered in conjunction with traditional weight-loss classes and counseling.

Loss of motivation is one of the leading causes of participant failure in a weight-loss program. Motivation can come from many sources, including the promise of reward, peer support, and competition. A team weight-loss competition combines these three strong motivators in a viable strategy to incorporate into a traditional weight-loss program.

Goals

To encourage reasonable and safe weight loss

To encourage a support system for weight-loss program participants

To provide motivation for participants to continue with a weight-loss program

Target audience

Although this competition could be offered to any adult audience, since participants must have frequent interaction with their team members, it is ideally suited to the workplace

Process

- Each team comprises four members. At the beginning of the contest each team member weighs in at the health promotion office and sets a weight-loss goal between one and ten pounds. The cap of ten pounds is set to discourage dangerous weight-loss practices.

  The teams have three months to achieve their weight loss goals. At the end of the three months, all teams must weigh in at the health promotion office.

  The winners are members of the team(s) that achieves the highest percentage of the cumulative weight-loss goal of all its members. For example, a group's total weight loss goal was 32 pounds, and the team members lost a total of 28 pounds, or 75 percent of their goal. One point is given for each percentage point, which in this case equals 75 points. (When calculating percentages, keep things simple. Round up for greater than 0.5 pounds and down for less than 0.5 pounds lost.)

No additional points are awarded for any individual weight lost in excess of the recorded goal.

Depending on the type of award being given to the winning team, in the event of a tie, the teams can split the award or receive matching awards, or the tying teams can determine an ultimate winner by drawing the winning team's name out of a hat.

- Besides organizing the competition, the health promotion staff should support the teams by

  providing weight-loss and other related classes during the three months of the competition;

  allowing participants to track their progress by weighing in at the health promotion office. Only the final weigh-in at the end of the competition is required.

- Encourage team members to support each other by

  frequently checking on one another's progress;

  exercising together;

  sharing dietary brown-bag lunches;

  attending weight-loss programs offered by the health promotion office together.

- Advertising for the program should

  encourage potential team members to form their own teams (the more the teams are made up of friends and coworkers, the more likely they are to see each other frequently and be supportive of each other during their weight loss efforts);

  commit the health promotion office to match up individuals who are not able to form a team;

  point out that since winning points are awarded based on the achieved percentage of weight-loss goal, all team members are equally competitive whether they want to lose one pound or ten pounds.

Cross-Reference: Chapter 36, Quick Tips (Healthy-heart pot luck/brown bag lunches)

38 Visual Illustrations of Food Content

Would you be less inclined to ask for a bacon cheeseburger if you could actually see the fat it contained? How about the sugar content in a big piece of pie? It probably would make you think twice. That is the logic behind this easy-to-construct display ideally suited for organizations with cafeterias or snack bars.

Typical hungry consumers do not pause to consider the nutritional value of the food they are about to eat. And if they did, the fat, sodium, and other nutritional measurements would be relatively meaningless to most. A visual illustration of food content gives consumers some idea of what they should (or should not) eat, to quickly and easily compare food choices prior to selection.

Goals

To educate consumers on healthy-heart eating

To encourage consumers to consider nutritional value of food when making selections

Target audience

All types

Process

- Choose the nutrition components to be highlighted:

  fat, sugar, or salt content

  recommended daily allowances of key nutrients
- Request copies of menus or nutrition labels from cafeteria or snack-bar food items to determine per-serving content of the highlighted components. In most cases, the nutritional information will be readily available from dining facility managers.
- To illustrate fat, sugar, or salt content, measure out the per-serving equivalent to the substance in small test tubes. To avoid constantly filling new test tubes for every meal, measure out a number of test tubes with varying amounts. Use a

compartmentalized box to store the test tubes not being used. Petroleum jelly works well to illustrate fat content, and any white powder can be used to illustrate salt or sugar content.

To avoid accidental spillage, seal the mouth of the test tubes with a cork or plastic wrap held in place by a rubber band.

- The two easiest ways to display the test tubes work equally well in most dining facility environments:

  Prominently display a menu board in the dining facility with the appropriate test tubes beside the day's menu selections. The test tubes can be labeled with the nutrient content being represented, or the menu board itself can state what the test tube contents represent.

  Place labeled test tubes on the glass in front of food selections in the serving line.

  If dining facility personnel are reliable, provide them with the appropriate test tubes for the day and ask them to change them with each meal.

- Illustrating such nutrients as vitamin C, calcium, protein, and the like, takes a little more ingenuity. It is probably best to highlight selected nutrients rather than all of them. The purpose of these visual illustrations is to encourage consumers to make selections of the food items with the greatest overall nutrient value. The following techniques allows the health promotion staff to reuse the same poster.

  Design the framework for a bar graph with the incremental measurements of the nutrients on sturdy poster board. Each bar graph represents the highlighted nutrient content for a menu item. For example, if vitamin C, calcium, protein, and calories are being highlighted, allow space for four bars and make a slit at the base of each bar. Label each bar with the name of the highlighted nutrient.

  Make as many posters as necessary to illustrate the total number of menu items to be analyzed daily. Place the name of the menu item on a separate piece of paper and attach either below or above the bars. Slip colored strips of sturdy paper or cloth the width and height of each bar through the slits from the back of the poster. Use a different color paper for each nutrient, but be consistent with the colors used on all the posters. Pull the bars (colored paper) through the slit to the appropriate height reflecting the content of the highlighted nutrient. Tape in place.

- Explain the intent of this nutrition initiative carefully. Today's dining facility personnel recognize the rising interest in healthy-heart eating. They will be more likely to provide the requested information and cooperate in displaying the test tubes and posters if reassured that customers will not be driven away.

- Initially, it is wise to have a health promotion manager present, at least during peak hours, to point out the test tubes and posters to consumers and explain their purpose.

Variation

Coordinate highlighting a single healthy-heart meal each day with dining facility managers. Visually display fat, salt, and/or sugar content as well as graphically display the nutrient content.

39 Healthy-Heart Cook-Offs

Healthy-heart food has gotten a "bad rap": it's bland, it's just rabbit food, and so on. Disprove the myths with healthy-heart cook-offs. Besides the obvious benefits, these cook-offs provide a great opportunity to get other wellness messages out. After all, as most health educators know, offer food and "they will come."

Many people have grown up cooking in a certain way and are reluctant to try unfamiliar techniques. People also cannot imagine that a food could taste good prepared any other way than the way they were taught. Past experience may have reinforced that idea. Many early attempts at healthy-heart cooking relied completely on boiling, broiling, and baking unseasoned food. Combining a competitive atmosphere with the prospect of sampling free or low-cost food is an excellent strategy to break this cycle of discomfort.

Goals

To illustrate that healthy food can taste good, as well as be good for you

To provide information on healthy-heart cooking techniques

To provide a forum for other health promotion information

Target audience

Adults

Process

- Contestants must register before the day of the contest in order for health promotion staff to counsel them on contest rules and healthy-heart cooking.

  Contestants have the option to cook a recipe of their own or to choose from recipes provided by the health promotion office. Recipes must comply with nutritional guidelines for healthy-heart eating provided by the health promotion office.

  If contestants are using their own recipes, they must give a copy to the health promotion staff before the contest for review and copying. Recipes that do not comply with required nutrition guidelines will not be allowed. If substitutions can be made to bring the recipe within nutrition guidelines, the health promotion staff can advise the contestant on the necessary changes. If the contestant agrees to the substitutions, the entry will be accepted.

- Depending on the anticipated size of the audience and whether they will be allowed to sample the entries,

  instruct the contestants on how many servings the entered food item must contain;

  in order to at least partially reimburse the contestants, consider charging a nominal cover charge for sampling the food items. A sampling cover charge can also be a fund-raising source for health promotion program incentives.
- Make the healthy-heart cook-offs an ongoing event. If the organization is large, rotate the responsibility for hosting the cook-off among departments or shifts. The health promotion staff provides the guidelines, but the sponsoring department provides the cooks and facility.
- If the healthy-heart cook-offs become an ongoing event, focus on a different type of food for each contest. A smorgasbord of different food items makes it difficult for the judges to decide on a winner. Suggestions for theme cook-offs:

  a particular category of food (soups, desserts, entrees, snacks, etc.)

  ethnic/cultural foods: Mexican, Italian, southern, etc.

  holiday/seasonal: Christmas, Thanksgiving, summer picnic/cookout, etc.
- Seek out well-known corporate managers, community leaders, or other dignitaries to act as judges for the contest. Include the names of the judges in the marketing campaign. Depending on the number of entries and size of the crowd, it may be best to have the judges make their decisions prior to the announced start of the program. Judging is based purely on the tastefulness of the food. Compliance with nutrition guidelines has already been determined.
- Provide handouts of each recipe or compile in a booklet for attendees.
- At the time of the judging, briefly explain to the attendees the nutrition criteria that were required in order to enter. Point out that healthy food can taste good! Once the judging has been accomplished and the awards have been given, allow attendees to sample the food.
- While attendees are eating, consider providing a short health promotion program.

Variation

Sponsor periodic healthy-heart cook-offs among dining facility cooks. This strategy is done on a smaller scale within the dining facility, but is meant to encourage dining facility staff to take a more active interest in nutrition. The winning cook receives an award, he or she is publicly recognized in the dining facility for customers to congratulate, and the winning entry is highlighted on the serving line for customers to try.

40 Inservices and Incentives for Snack Bar Personnel

Health educators are always looking for the teachable moment. Such moments occur virtually every day as people go through cafeteria lines. Line servers can be a great resource. All you need is to give them a little attention, a little education, and some motivation. This chapter gives you some very workable ideas.

Dining facility personnel underestimate the impact they have on the health of their customers. Customers going through a serving line are receptive to nutrition information. Being able to rely on dining facility personnel to answer simple questions and to know where to refer customers with more complex questions is an invaluable asset to the health promotion manager.

Goals

To educate dining facility personnel on nutrition

To motivate dining facility personnel to take an active interest in enhancing the nutrition status of their customers

Target audience

Directly: cafeteria or snack-bar personnel

Indirectly: customers of the cafeteria or snack bar

Process

- Determine the nutrition training of dining facility personnel.
- Offer to conduct a series of nutrition/healthy eating inservices to address any deficit areas in their education. Provide videotapes and other learning tools that can be used during staff breaks.
- In addition to the inservices, provide a nutrition tip to the staff frequently (at least weekly, if not daily). The "tip" can be provided during staff meetings or in the form of a poster. Besides nutrition information, inservices and tips should include information on where customers can be referred to get more advanced nutrition counseling or other more sophisticated information.

- Once the inservice training is underway, initiate an ongoing dining facility staff competition. The purpose of the competition is to test dining facility personnel on key information provided in the inservices.

  Periodically, a "planted" customer asks a nutrition-related question randomly of a server while going through the line at a mealtime. This question should be somewhat challenging and should refer to information that would be useful to the server in answering real customer questions and making decisions that affect the nutritional value of the food.

  Preferably, this question is asked at a busy time of the day, when customers can benefit from the information and congratulate the server (assuming he or she can answers the question correctly).

  If the dining facility staff member correctly answers the question, a health promotion staff member (or other designated official) who was discreetly standing by comes forward and congratulates the server and gives him or her an incentive award or prize.

  If the dining facility staff member cannot answer the question, to avoid embarrassing the server, the "planted" customer quietly hands him or her a card with the question and correct answer, then moves on through the line without comment.

- Promote the dining facility staff's cooperation and new expertise in nutrition counseling to the customers. Encourage them to visit the cafeteria or snack bar and ask questions.

Variation

Once the dining facility personnel education program has been completed, offer the cafeteria and snack-bar personnel the opportunity to take a voluntary nutrition test. If they successfully pass the test, provide them with a designation that sets them above the other line servers as a basic nutrition counselor. Give them a pin that reflects this title. For instance: "Certified by your Health Promotion Office as a "'Cafeteria Nutrition Counselor.'" Encourage customers to seek out these people.

Cross-Reference: Chapter 38, Visual Illustrations of Food Content

41 Label-Reading Contests

Grocery shopping is another of those teachable moments health educators love. Participating shoppers search for a food item that best meets criteria established by the health promotion staff. Offer the contest often. Just change the criteria and watch valuable label-reading habits get used more and more.

Most grocery store food selections are influenced by advertising, shelf placement, or the lowest price. Label reading is rarely a factor. It takes an external motivator to change this shopping behavior.

Goals

To encourage customers to read food labels

To educate customers on nutrition

Target audience

Adults

Process

- The label-reading contest is a series of contests run in a grocery store. The contest

  encourages participants to compare labels of a specific category of food products (e.g., cereal, bread, TV entrées, crackers, package mixes, baby food, ice cream, margarine, etc.);

  defines criteria for selecting the best food product(s) (the criteria can be one or more of any of the following nutrients: salt; sugar; total fat, saturated fat, monounsaturated fat, polyunsaturated fats; simple versus complex carbohydrates (dietary fiber); protein; cholesterol; specific vitamins; calcium; iron;

  defines serving size in the criteria (not all food product serving sizes are the same).

  To be fair, contestants can only bring one food item at a time to the health promotion staff for evaluation.

- Advance marketing of this contest is important for maximum participation, but the type of marketing done will depend on the target audience of the sponsoring health promotion program.

- At least one health promotion staff member needs to be present in the grocery store for the duration of the contests to

  explain contest rules;

  hand out informational brochures explaining the importance of the highlighted nutrient and any calculations that need to be done;

  answer questions;

  evaluate food products brought up by customers, to determine the winner.

  Determining contest winners will be expedited if the health promotion staff has already evaluated most or all of the food products ahead of time. The staff member should be ready to explain to customers why their selections are not the best choices.

- Marketing should reflect the starting time of the first contest, but indicate that a series of contests will be run throughout the day until a certain time. Customers can enter a contest at any time while the contest is running. An individual contest is concluded and a winner declared when the correct product is found. A single contest per day can be run, but a daylong series of contests generates more interest.

- Consider making a display of the food categories being highlighted for each contest. Each display should show

  what the criteria are for the contest;

  why choosing food products that meet these criteria is important;

  how to determine the nutrient content from the product label.

  At the end of each contest, add the food item(s) meeting the defined criteria to the display.

- One strategy for obtaining contest incentives or prizes is to approach vendors of products that best meet the contest criteria. Since their products are being highlighted, vendors may be very open to providing free or discount coupons.

Cross-Reference: Chapter 46, Grocery Store Scavenger Hunt

42 Cholesterol Clinics

It is not enough for clients to "know their (cholesterol) numbers." They must understand what the information means and what to do with it. This clinic concept appeals to the audience's natural desire to "know their numbers," but is structured to encourage attendance at a variety of coronary artery risk-reduction programs while being tested.

Cholesterol screening with minimal follow-up counseling and education leaves audiences without the necessary tools to take action to lower their coronary artery risks. Such audiences tend to view cholesterol screening as they would a blood-pressure check or weigh-in and have cholesterol tests at inappropriately frequent intervals. Cholesterol tests without a health care provider recommendation are meaningless and a waste of resources.

Goals

To enable audiences with hypercholesterolemia to control their coronary artery risks

To maximize the effectiveness of cholesterol screening resources

Target audience

Primarily adults with elevated cholesterol

Process

- Coordinate with a cooperating laboratory, wellness center, or other appropriate source for interested audiences to access a first-time cholesterol screening.
- Provide the cholesterol screening locations with prepared instructions for participants on how to obtain test results:

  Participants must attend a cholesterol education class to get their cholesterol results. Allow no exceptions. So they do not have to wait an inordinate amount of time, offer the class on an ongoing basis every two weeks. (At a minimum, offer the class once a month.) When they are tested, participants should automatically be scheduled for the follow-up program. Inform them of the class date and time. Impress on the client that attendance is expected.

- The initial cholesterol education class provides general information on cholesterol, other coronary artery risks, and their interrelated role in heart disease and strokes. Explain what the cholesterol test numbers mean and how each individual should interpret the results. Since many questions will be common among participants, dedicate plenty of time for a class question-answer period.
- Individuals with cholesterol elevations warranting follow-up are given access to one-on-one consultations, other programs, and referrals at the end of the class. A staff member should be available with a health care provider, dietitian, and program schedules to set up appointments on the spot.
- If follow-up appointments verify that an individual with a cholesterol elevation needs monitoring, he or she is automatically enrolled in the cholesterol clinic.

  Offer a follow-up screening and education class every three months. (Depending on audience size, it may be necessary to offer these programs twice a quarter.)

  Participants are automatically scheduled for each three-month session when they attend the previous class. They are given an appointment slip and sent a one-week reminder prior to each session. Emphasize that their attendance is treated like a doctor's appointment. This improves compliance and attendance.
- Each quarterly session(s) offers a class on some aspect of coronary artery risk reduction. Examples:

  the low fat diet

  role of fitness in reducing cardiac risks

  importance of controlling other health risks such as smoking, blood pressure, diabetes, etc.

  A new topic is offered every three months. Since new participants will be entering the clinic throughout the year, each topic should not be dependent on previous lectures, but should be complementary to them.
- Participants receive a cholesterol test as each lecture is presented.

  Set up a blood-drawing station in a corner of the lecture room. Put up a screen, if necessary, to provide privacy but still allow individuals to listen to the presentation. If the station is at the back of the room, behind the participants, then a screen may not be necessary, and participants can see the lecture as well.

  Ideally, health promotion staff members can fill out laboratory slips prior to each session, based on participant information provided during registration at the class in the previous quarter. But if necessary, before beginning the lecture explain how to fill out the laboratory slips and let participants quietly fill them out while waiting for the lecture to begin.

Tell participants the sequence in which they will go to the blood-drawing station, for example, starting at the back of the room and moving right to left on each aisle. Each person can automatically go in when the person prior to him or her comes out, without disturbing the lecture.

- The results of the laboratory tests are forwarded to each individual's health care provider. Providers are responsible for notifying their patients and making whatever recommendations are appropriate.
- Keep a record for participants, showing when they had blood tests and what programs they attended. Copies of the record should be forwarded to the participants' health care providers.

Maternal/Child Programming

43 Quick Tips

Bring them up right! These high-impact, low-cost quick tips help you to help kids learn about wellness, nutrition, emotional health, and more.

■ **Wellness story hour**

Search libraries and bookstores for children's books dealing with health and wellness topics, or write your own stories. Approach day care centers, libraries, and schools and offer to read to the children there. Put on a costume or bring puppets and act out the stories. Provide a recommended reading list of wellness stories to childcare givers.

■ **"Touchy-feely" box**

The "touchy-feely" box is a children's teaching aid about the sense of touch. Decorate a box large enough to contain items no bigger than a volleyball. Cut a hole in the side about three to four inches in diameter. Tape or glue a small piece of cloth to cover the hole from the inside. It should be possible to open the box to put small items inside. Use various objects with distinct tactile qualities, such as chilled or heated gel packs, unusually shaped furry toys, a pumice stone, Silly Putty, and more. A child places his or her hand in the hole of the box, finds the object, and describes it through touch. Encourage the child to be aware of which parts of the hand is most sensitive to the different sensations.

■ **"Kick the habit"**

As a break activity during a presentation on substance abuse, hang a heavy boot from a rope. Set up large models of cigarettes, drugs, or alcohol. Make a game of trying to kick the drugs and knock them over.

■ **Build a food pyramid**

After explaining the nutritional food pyramid, draw the framework of a giant food pyramid on butcher paper or poster board. Using plastic food models, make a game to see who can get the correct foods in the proper quadrant of the pyramid in the shortest period of time.

■ **Posture obstacle course**

Construct a simple obstacle course (outside or inside) that involves mostly walking, and if possible, a few steps to climb and/or descend. Each child places a beanbag on his or her head. The winner of the game is the first child to navigate the course without the beanbag falling off.

■ **"Fix the people"**

As part of a basic anatomy class, challenge kids to find the correct organ based on finding the answer to two riddles. Using an anatomical mannequin, put the body parts in their proper place as each set of riddles is answered. Each riddle provides a different clue to the organ and its function. For instance, (1) I have been known to run on occasions; (2) some people would not see well without me: the nose (runs when you have a cold, and glasses would not stay up).

■ **"Warm fuzzies"**

Ask a group of kids how they feel when they say something nice about someone else. Most kids will say they feel good about themselves. How do they feel when someone says something nice about them? Of course, that makes them feel good. If we feel good . . . and they feel good . . . why don't we say nice things about others more often? Discuss the reasons; then say, "Well, let's make up for all those missed opportunities." Tape a piece of paper on each child's back. The kids then walk around with felt-tip pens writing something nice about the others on their backs. Remind the kids they can say nice things and funny things, but no hurtful things. Tell the kids no one will know who wrote the "warm fuzzies" since the kids won't get to read them until later. The anonymity should help overcome their natural shyness. At the end of the activity, kids can volunteer to read their "warm fuzzies" if they want to, but it is not required.

■ **Punching bags**

Everyone gets angry occasionally. Help children develop positive strategies for channeling their anger. Ask each child to think of something that makes them really angry, then start punching on the bag. Soon they will be laughing. Explain that physical activity helps anger go away harmlessly without hurting anyone. As a group, discuss situations where they may get angry and different ways to use other types of physical activity to calm down.

■ **Stress balloons**

In a group setting, each child fills a balloon with flour. Keep the size small enough so the balloon can be handled easily and squeezed by little hands. Tie off the ends. Talk to the kids about feeling anxious. Tell them they can control how bad these feelings make them feel. Their balloon is a special toy for making anxious feelings go away. They squeeze and play with the toy until they are feeling better.

■ **Local bodybuilder superhero(ines)**

Seek volunteers from among local bodybuilders to become wellness superheroes (or heroines). Accentuate already buffed bodies with a superhero costume (a leotard, giant "W" for "Wellness (Wo)Man," and cape will do in a pinch) and off they go to do battle with "Fat Monsters," "Mr. Tooth Decay," "Couch Potatoes," "Red Rage Monsters," and other types of wellness adversaries. The health promotion manager discusses the message, while the superhero keeps the kids' attention. Work with the volunteers so that they may eventually teach the message themselves.

■ **Bigotry lessons**

Help kids discover the truth behind bigotry and get a taste of what it feels like to be a maligned minority. The children think of a number of physical features some people might share, but others don't, for example, freckles, blue eyes, long hair, left-handedness. Place slips of paper with each of the features into a hat and draw one out. Whatever the feature, declare that for the next hour (two hours, day, etc.); we are not going to like anyone with that characteristic. Discuss with the children how they can demonstrate they don't like that type of person. Acknowledge that they could physically hurt them, but emphasize that it will not be allowed. The students return to their normal activities. Periodically remind them to dislike the children with the unfortunate feature. At the end of the designated period of time, gather the kids to discuss how they felt as they picked on children with that feature, how did the children being picked on feel, and finally whether disliking someone for something so superficial really makes sense. End the lesson by saying, "Now of course, we really don't hate anyone" and having a special group hug for any of the children who were being harassed. As time allows, repeat this activity, choosing different characteristics so that eventually everyone is a member of the targeted minority.

■ **Trampoline aerobic demonstration**

Demonstrate the impact of exercise on heart health. Set up a trampoline. Let the children listen to the heart rate of one or more children. If possible, use a Doppler to project the heartbeat for everyone to hear at once. Explain the importance of exercise for heart health. Ask the child(ren) to jump on the trampoline for five minutes, then take the heart rate again. Depending on the age and comprehension level of the children, discussion can go into recovery time and include listening to the heart at intervals until it returns to normal.

- **Healthy pet program**

Ask a local veterinarian or representative from a petting zoo to bring in two or three tame animals of different species. Ask the guest to highlight topics of pet health that parallel wellness messages about people: care of the teeth, proper diet, sufficient rest, care of the hair/fur, exercise, immunizations, and so on. Give equal time to the guest speaker discussing the animal health issues, then the health promotion manager tying his or her comments into wellness messages for people.

- **Preggy pillows**

Designed to simulate the weight and appearance of an advanced pregnancy, this teaching aid is worn for prolonged periods of time to allow girls to begin to appreciate the not-so-glamorous aspects of pregnancy: body image, back aches, altered center of gravity, even personal hygiene become new challenges. The preggy pillow can be a useful teaching aid for boys, as well.

- **Raising baby (doll)**

A programmable baby doll teaches girls and boys that babies aren't always cute and cuddly. The baby demands to be fed, changed, rocked, and even then isn't always satisfied. A useful tool to deglamorize teen pregnancy.

- **Seat-belt safety**

Jeeps can be rolled with relatively little damage to the vehicle. Use mannequins or other types of dummies to illustrate the results on the human body of an automobile accident. Have an experienced driver (wearing a seat belt and helmet) roll the jeep in a field with the dummies first wearing, and then not wearing, seat belts.

- **Tobacco-cessation shock therapy**

Many health educators who work with adolescents and teens will verify that they want to be shocked, especially when it applies to the hazards of smoking. Take teen tobacco-cessation or awareness classes to oncology wards or intensive care units. Ask nurses if any patients suffering from tobacco-related illness would be willing to talk to the students. Ask doctors to explain some of the procedures they must employ in their attempts to prolong the lives of cancer patients.

- **Parent-child weight-training program**

Market a weight-training program targeting parents and teenagers. The training includes proper techniques in the use of free weights, as well as how to coach and spot for a partner. Besides the fitness benefits of this program, feedback from these programs indicates enhanced parent-child communication in other aspects of the relationship.

School physicals

Take advantage of school physicals to reach younger audiences. There is a lot of standing-around time in clinics during school physicals. Reach these younger audiences through wellness videos and games. Conduct needs assessments and surveys of the kids and their parents.

Cross-Reference: Section 8, Resources

44 Baby Aerobics

After the initial glow of a new baby's birth wanes, what do many mothers worry about? Getting their figure back. The Baby Aerobics program brings new mothers together to exercise with their babies. It provides the necessary aerobic benefit, a great mother/baby bonding experience, and creates a natural support system for new mothers.

Unwanted weight gain resulting from pregnancy is a well-known problem for newly delivered mothers. Many women point to difficulty in finding child care, the cost of child care, or a reluctance to place young infants in a child-care environment as an obstacle to exercise. The Baby Aerobics program removes all of these obstacles and has the added advantage of creating an automatic support group for new mothers.

Goals

To assist new mothers in losing any unwanted weight

To encourage maternal/child bonding

To encourage formation of a new-mother support group

Target audience

New mothers with infants under one year

Process

- A fitness specialist should develop an aerobics program that focuses primarily on the legs. It is important to keep the center of gravity stable since the exercising mothers hold their babies throughout the program. Minimize jumping, lunging, and other movements that could unbalance the mother and cause her to fall or drop the baby.
- Floor activities can be done with the mother holding the infant on her stomach or laying the infant in front of her.
- While most of the exercise routine should be done with the legs, some activity can include moving the baby with the arms (rocking, holding the baby out from the

body, up in the air, etc.). The aerobic benefit of the entire exercise routine will be enhanced by the baby's weight.

- Choose a location and exercise time(s) that is least likely to disturb other activities not involving children, while accommodating a group of women with infants.
- Have a diaper-changing area available.
- Encourage the new mothers in the class to socialize with each other. Part of the value for the Baby Aerobics program is the therapeutic interaction of women with infants of comparable ages.
- Advertise the Baby Aerobics program through obstetricians, pediatricians, family practitioners, obstetric wards, and other resources for new mothers.

45 Mothers' Club

Provide a support system for first-time expectant mothers through the intervention of experienced and trained volunteer mothers. Club mothers are assigned immediately on the birth of the child, while the new mother is still in the hospital, and continue into the home for as long as necessary.

Whether it's a result of geographic separation or a breakdown of the family unit, young first-time mothers and their babies lacking a reliable support system are at increased risk emotionally and physically. With proper oversight and training, experienced volunteer mothers can create a supportive environment for these women and children.

Goals

To promote mother/child bonding

To assist new mothers' development of child-rearing skills

To make the early identification of high-risk family environments

To encourage appropriate use of the health care system

Target audience

First-time, inexperienced new mothers; especially effective for teenagers and women in their early 20s

Process

- Seek Mothers' Club volunteers through these sources:

  local newspapers and organizations whose target audience includes women with experience in raising children

  pediatricians and family practitioners

  women's clubs

  day-care centers

  elementary schools

senior citizen centers

churches

- Establish an orientation for Mothers' Club volunteers. Discuss club policies on issues such as

    appropriate interaction with new mothers;

    limits to advice/assistance that may be offered;

    professional backup personnel/agencies.

  If possible, partner a new volunteer with an experienced volunteer to observe before allowing her to work with a new mother on her own.

- Identify sources for referral of candidates for Mothers' Club services. Examples:

  obstetric health care providers

  hospital obstetric units

  social services

  department of public health

- Provide referral sources with information and briefings on the Mothers' Club, including these factors:

  goals and objectives

  policies

  training and oversight of volunteers

  background of professional staff who manage volunteers

  names and phone numbers of those to contact when potential candidates in need of club services are identified

- Compile a reference list of agencies that may provide assistance to new mothers, and acquaint all Mothers' Club volunteers with the list. Examples:

  United Way

  social services

  department of public health

  child and family counselors

  local hospitals, clinics, emergency rooms

- Establish an on-call schedule so referral agencies know which Mothers' Club members to contact for services.

Seek to have a club member visit the new mother within twenty-four hours after a request. Initiate the relationship with the new mother as soon after the birth as possible, preferably while the mother is still in the hospital.

The same club member should be assigned to a new mother until services are no longer needed or are terminated.

- Avoid burnout among the club members:

  Track how many new mothers a club member is assigned to.

  Let members decide how many hours they want to volunteer per month.

  Recognize that a new mother will be more demanding in the first few weeks after birth, and stagger assignments accordingly.

- Provide a list of health care providers who agree to make themselves available for telephone consultation with Mothers' Club volunteers encountering problems they don't know how to deal with.

- Services/benefits for the new mother:

  assistance in developing simple child-care skills, such as diapering, bathing, feeding/burping

  assistance in setting up the baby's room and other aspects of modifying the home for the new baby

  reassurance and advice: (ideally, volunteer mothers should make themselves available at any time for telephone consultation.)

  The Mothers' Club should not be used as a baby-sitting service, but club members can use their discretion to relieve mothers for short periods of time under unique circumstances.

- Require club mothers to attend periodic meetings, including programs on topics dealing with child rearing through the first year and other challenges facing the new mother. Examples:

  postpartal depression: what is it, how to deal with it, when to seek help

  choosing child care

  normal growth and development

  home treatments for minor illnesses and injuries and signs that medical attention is needed breast-feeding, weaning, introducing solids, milk intolerance, etc.

crying: what does it mean, how to keep it from getting to you

childproofing the home

Meetings should include cross-talk on real-life problems encountered by volunteers in working with assigned mothers/families.

Meetings should be facilitated by a health care professional experienced in parenting issues.

- As a rule, Mothers' Club members should begin to disengage themselves from a new mother at around six months after birth, but no later than a year. New mothers should understand that this is part of club policy.

  Encourage new mothers to provide a critique and feedback on services at time of disengagement.

- Note: There is an added side-benefit for some volunteer mothers. Stay-at-home mothers whose children have moved out and are on their own sometimes wonder what they can still contribute to society. The Mothers' Club offers a wonderful opportunity for these women to build self-confidence and to enrich and improve others' lives.

46 Grocery Store Scavenger Hunt

Get kids to start reading labels! Impossible, you say; but with this field trip to the local grocery store, that's exactly what they will do. As in the old party game, kids search for food products that meet the defined criteria on their "scavenger hunt" shopping list.

Children are strongly influenced by advertising. While one game will not change teenagers into smart shoppers, combined with an appropriate education program, it will begin to influence their decisions.

Goals

To encourage preteens and teens to begin reading food labels

To educate preteens and teens on nutrition

Target audience

Ten to fifteen preteens and teenagers

Process

- Hold the grocery store scavenger hunt in a supermarket with adult supervision. It is not necessary for other patrons to stop shopping, although it may be advisable to hold back traffic in the area at the start of the race.

  Approach a local grocery store with the concept. Ask them what times they would prefer the contest be run to avoid inconveniencing patrons. There will be some natural concerns about having so many teens and adolescents in their store at once. Discuss the precautions listed in this chapter, but also emphasize the promotional benefits:

  advertising to all the parents as well as the school staff

  increased business: many of the parents and teachers present for the contest will likely do some shopping there and may become repeat customers

  increased goodwill for a store that so obviously supports the wellness program

- Offer nutrition classes to the participants through their schools or youth centers.

Include in the opening remarks to the class, as well as any marketing, an explanation of the upcoming competition. Stress that class attendees will be better able to win the scavenger hunt by listening closely to the information in the program.

- The contest challenges participants to find as many food items as possible from a scavenger hunt list of criteria developed by the health promotion staff. Choose the criteria carefully:

  Specify categories of food versus seasonings, package mixes, and other food items that would not be of interest to this audience.

  Avoid food items that may be easily damaged from handling.

  Make it necessary for the participants to read the label.

  Highlight important nutrients. For each of the following nutrients, require scavengers to look for an item that meets at least 50 percent of the RDA: vitamin C, calcium, or iron.

  Point participants toward healthy choices they can include in their everyday diets:

    a fat-free and sugar-free candy, a nonmeat food item with at least 1 percent protein, a food item that is at least 24 percent dietary fiber.

  Define serving size (not all food product serving sizes are the same).

- Participants are given a grocery cart for gathering the items on their scavenger hunt list.
- Rules should stipulate safe operation of the grocery carts and careful handling of food (broken or damaged items will not count towards winning, and the contestant may be required to buy the item if damage was from recklessness).
- At least one health promotion staff member with a nutrition background needs to be present in the grocery store to

  explain the contest rules;

  hand out informational brochures explaining the importance of the highlighted nutrients and any calculations that need to be done;

  answer questions;

  advise other staff members and volunteers;

  evaluate food products gathered by the contestants to determine the winner.

Additional adult supervision from other health promotion staff, volunteers, or store personnel will be needed to

monitor the aisles as the hunt progresses;

assist in evaluating food products brought up by the contestants;

help return the food items to their appropriate places after the contest concludes.

- Anticipate a number of parents being present for the scavenger hunt. Use this as a teachable moment to discuss the importance of label reading and the nutrients being highlighted.
- Consider making a display about the scavenger hunt. Each display should show

  criteria for the contest;

  the importance of choosing food products that meet these criteria;

  how to determine the nutrient content from the product label.

  At the end of the contest, display a sampling of the food items meeting the defined criteria.
- Have at least one award for the individual who gathers the most food items that best meet the criteria on the list. Depending on resources, consider a first, second, and third place award.

  Runner-up incentives can come from free or discount coupons for products that best meet the criteria listed on the list. Since their products are being highlighted, vendors may be very open to providing coupons.

Cross-Reference: Chapter 41, Label-Reading Contests

47 Grocery Bag Art Contests

Let kids get out your wellness messages. Sponsor a health promotion art contest using paper grocery bags from local stores for the canvas. Then recycle all of the "art work" back to the store when the contest is over. Shoppers, as well as the kids, will get the message.

Children learn through doing. Teach a child a simple lesson, then ask him to draw a picture of what was learned. The lesson will stay with the child much longer. Adults learn from children. The simplicity of a child's picture or question cuts through all the rationalizations erected by adults.

Goals

To raise awareness of wellness concepts in adults and children

To stimulate interest in the health promotion program

Target audience

Elementary-school children

Process

- Grocery bag art contests differ from traditional children's art contest in only one way: the "canvases" for the drawings are paper grocery bags. Choose any nontoxic medium, although to avoid smearing, the less greasy the better.
- Approach a local grocery store and request donations of their paper grocery bags for use in a health promotion art contest. Emphasize that most of the grocery bags will be returned after the art contest with children's wellness messages drawn on each. They are encouraged to use the returned bags with the artwork.

  As a result of the grocery bag contributions, the store will receive positive publicity for their support of the program, as well as the interest generated by new customers coming to the store to shop and get a child's submission on a grocery bag.
- Approach day-care centers or elementary schools to encourage participation.
- The art contest can focus on a specific health topic or encourage general wellness messages.

- To kick off the art contest, conduct a program illustrating the types of messages that are the goal of the contest.
- Each student receives one grocery bag. Although students should be discouraged from using a number of bags before completing their projects, it is realistic to expect some waste. Provide a few extras to the adults supervising the children as they draw.
- Judging of the art contests can be done in any way desired by the health promotion staff to meet the goals of the program. Give first, second, and third place awards. Give awards for different age ranges if appropriate.
- Once the contest is over, all grocery bags go back to the grocery store and are placed in the checkout lanes for normal use. The winning bag(s) can be displayed at the front of the store to encourage customers to ask for paper bags in the checkout line. To encourage use of the bags, baggers can ask, "Do you want plastic or a piece of art?"

48 Circulation Game

Kids understand the circulatory system and consequences of hardening of the arteries by actually being involved in the circulation process. A few easy-to-obtain materials and a little floor space are all you need.

The more children are involved in the learning process, the more they will retain the important elements of a wellness message. It is never too soon to begin teaching children basic concepts about their bodies and how their personal choices can effect long-term health.

Goals

To lay the groundwork for heart-healthy attitudes and behaviors in children

Target audience

Ten or more preschool and elementary-age children

Process

- The Circulation Game is a group activity that requires the following accessories:

  a large bulb syringe or turkey baster to represent the heart's pumping action: fill it with water;

  red construction paper cut into a series of circles approximately ten inches in diameter: the red circles can be pinned onto a child's chest, or staple the middle of a string to the center of the red circle so a child can wear the circle on their head;

  approximately four large white sheets sewn together: draw a basic schematic of the heart and major vessels on the sheets with indelible ink. It is not important for the schematic to be anatomically correct; rather it should be a simple representation of cardiac circulation. Draw a picture of an ear near the end of the artery representing circulation to the head and a picture of a foot with an enlarged big toe near the artery representing the circulation to the body. The arteries should be wide enough to allow two or three small children to pass through close together;

  approximately four standard-sized pillows and belts.

- Before the first part of the game, explain to the children that

  the heart is a pump that pushes blood through the body (use the bulb syringe to demonstrate the heart contracting and pushing blood—the water—out through the aorta);

  the blood is important for carrying food to the toes and their ears and everything in between;

  it is important for the tubes carrying the blood to be nice and big and smooth so the blood can get where it needs to go.

- The game, part 1: If the heart schematic is going to be used more than once, it might be a good idea to have the children take off their shoes. This also will minimize any discomfort from stepped-on toes or accidental kicking.

  Line up three or four children along each side of the artery wall leading from the heart. The children link hands and now represent the artery. If the schematic is big enough and there are enough children, have children represent artery walls going to both the head and the body.

  Pin or tie red circles on three or four children, who now represent the blood cells. If circulation to the head and feet is represented and there are enough children, double the number of children who represent blood cells and show them which artery path to take. Tell the children that they are now carrying food to the ears and the toes along nice smooth healthy arteries.

  Gather all the "blood cells" in the heart at the entrance to the artery. The instructor holds his or her arms wide apart as if to embrace the children and says, "I am playing the heart. I am getting ready to pump you out into the arteries. When I bring my arms together, out you go!" The instructor comes towards the kids, steadily bringing his or her arms together, and herds them out into the artery.

  The artery-wall children merely hold hands, and the blood cell players can walk quickly through the vessels from the heart and out the end. The arteries should be wide enough to allow this without problem. The artery players can lean back a little if it is necessary to let the blood cells through. Explain that healthy arteries are limber (like a piece of spaghetti or similar analogy) and give a little when blood is pumped through and that they then return to their normal shape when the heart is resting.

- Before the second part of the game, explain to the children that

  eating too much fatty food and not enough healthy food slowly, but surely, leaves a waxy film on the inside of the artery walls that makes it increasingly difficult for the blood to move through them;

  if the ears, toes, and other parts of the body do not get as much food as they should, they will not be as healthy as they should be;

  eventually some of these vessels may be blocked altogether, and the parts of the body fed by those arteries don't get any food from the blood at all, this blockage can even make the heart less healthy.

- The game, part 2:

  Tie the pillows around the waists of the artery children. This represents the waxy buildup of arteriosclerosis. Also tell the artery players to try not to lean back this time as the blood tries to go through. Explain how the waxy buildup not only makes the arteries narrower, but makes them stiffer too. They cannot expand as much when the heart pushes the blood through.

  The instructor again gathers the children in the heart and simulates a heartbeat.

  The children try to move quickly through the artery. This should be much more difficult now. If they "blood cells" get stuck altogether, explain that this is how an artery get blocked: the blood can't get through.

- Conclude the game by discussing things the children can do to keep their arteries nice and clean. While it is important to reduce fats, at this age children need more fats than adults; so do not overemphasize this area. Rather, focus on eating more healthy foods, such as fruits and vegetables, reducing snacks like candy, and exercising.

Variation

Relay races: Each team is composed of one child wearing a red circle to represent oxygenated blood and carrying a balloon filled with air and a banana (or similar healthy food), and another child wearing a blue circle to represent blood cells that have given up their food and oxygen to cells and carrying a small wastebasket to represent the waste products from the cells.

The race starts with all the red cells at the heart (home base) and each deoxygenated cell standing by a picture of a body part (ear, toe, etc.) at equal distances from the heart. Each red cell races from the heart to the deoxygenated cell with the balloon and banana, and tags the deoxygenated blood cell, who then runs back to the heart, carrying the wastebasket.

A similar relay race can be done to demonstrate pulmonary circulation. The blue cells run to the lungs with deflated balloons, and the red cells run back with inflated balloons.

Programs and Activities for Healthy Aging

49 Programs and Activities for the Stages of Life

We may stop growing when we become adults; but for men and women alike, every stage of adulthood presents unique physical and emotional changes. These changes do not stop until the day we die. This chapter suggests ideas for healthy-aging programs, which are sure to increase the appeal of any wellness program.

Much of the fear of aging comes from myths perpetuated by the media and American culture. Even the medical profession adds to misperceptions about healthy aging. How often have we heard doctors brush off aging patients' complaints of an ache or pain with comments like "Oh, that just comes with growing old"? In fact, many of the common ailments previously accepted as natural to the aging process can be prevented or minimized. And since we will all face the inevitable prospect of our own or a loved one's death, a healthy attitude about this final stage of life will add quality to those last days as well.

Target audience

All types, middle-age and older

Goals

To provide strategies for adapting to the normal physical, mental, and emotional changes of aging

To minimize preventable physical, mental, and emotional deterioration

To provide information on, and facilitate access to, available community services for senior citizens

Process

- Make sure the facility is fully accessible to people who use wheelchairs or have physical limitations.
- Programming ideas:

  general health-risk assessments and topic-specific assessments: coronary artery risks, fitness, stress, nutrition, etc.

general self-care for older audiences: hair loss, menopause, hormone replacement, skin changes, hearing changes, constipation, bone density, changing libido

self-care for health problems common to the aging: Alzheimer's disease, Parkinson's disease, arthritis, diabetes, coronary artery disease, bunions/hammertoes, cataracts, glaucoma, gout, circulatory problems, incontinence, leg pain, prostate problems, weakness/fatigue

sexuality

changing nutrition needs: strategies for meeting these needs in people with decreasing appetites, dos and don'ts of supplements

importance of a regular fitness program

adjusting to widow(er)hood

strategies for staying mentally alert

death and dying: physical and mental changes as the end nears, stages of grief, how to be supportive to a dying friend/loved one, legal considerations, what to do after the death (funerals, personal effects, notifying family, newspaper announcements, etc.)

- Periodic screening services:

  blood chemistries for coronary artery disease

  gout and renal function

  blood pressure

  blood glucose

  dental

  foot checks and nail trimming

  skin cancer

  Pap smears

  prostate

  breast exams and mammograms

  colorectal cancer

Cross-Reference: Chapter 23, Senior Fairs; Chapter 50, Programs and Activities for Encouraging Independence and Safety; Chapter 51, Programs and Activities for Staying Connected; Section 8, Resources

50 Programs and Activities for Encouraging Independence and Safety

Personal safety is of primary concern to any adult, especially today. These concerns become more profound in the later years, as maintaining one's typical activities of daily living become increasingly difficult. This chapter suggests programs to meet this very basic need.

The biggest obstacle to independence for older people is the difficulty of convincing them that they do have control over their lives. Once that is accomplished, other factors seem much less daunting. Decreasing strength, flexibility, and vitality will probably be a reality for everyone at some point in their lives. However, when that point is reached, and the degree to which it limits an individual, can be influenced. Many of the benefits of healthy lifestyles can be felt even when the individual begins late in life. While other issues such as crime and money are very real concerns, there are resources to help.

Goals

To increase the self-confidence of older audiences

To assist older audiences in maintaining their personal safety

Target audience

All types, middle-age and older

Process

- Make sure the facility is fully accessible to people who use wheelchairs or have physical limitations.
- Programming ideas:

  discussion of the options to living alone: assisted-living facilities, retirement homes, living with family, professional/semiprofessional at-home caregivers

  medication awareness programs: discussing over-the-counter medications, prescription medications, changing medication needs with age, drug/drug interactions; include opportunities for audiences to have their prescription and over-the-counter medications and supplements analyzed for compatibility

self-defense training and self-defense equipment

fighting crimes against the aging

elder abuse, intimidation, robbery at home and on the streets

home safety strategies:

to prevent break-ins: outside lights, security systems, locking systems, neighborhood watch programs, etc.

to prevent falls and other accidents: securing rugs, rails, lifting equipment

to expedite responses to accidents: personal electronic response systems, community emergency response systems, volunteer programs to check on the old and infirm

telephone scams: identifying, resisting, reporting

assertiveness programs

cooking classes (especially for men)

being an active participant in one's own health care

exercise classes to increase strength, endurance, and mobility

mature driving programs: designed to help older drivers adjust driving techniques to diminished response times, vision, flexibility, etc.

retirement and personal finances, which are major concerns and sources of stress for this population:

financial health: include goal setting and orienting the use of "all" money toward a values-based financial plan

preparing to retire: developing a concrete vision of what retirement life should be, testing that vision (what will be given up as well as gained), and developing a plan to make the vision a reality

adjusting to retirement: role adjustments, decreased income

updates on changes in Medicare and the Social Security system

- Other programs and services:

form/support local programs, such as neighborhood watch, organizations or volunteers to check on "shut-ins" and the infirm, escort programs to the store, medical appointments, etc., Meals on Wheels;

provide a senior massage service: besides the well-known therapeutic value of massage, a number of specialized massage techniques help optimize mobility for seniors and minimize many of the problems encountered in the later years. Areas that can be specifically helped by these massage techniques include peripheral vascular disease, foot deformities and gait problems, lymphedema, stiff neck, backs, and joints, arthritis, facial "masking" from Parkinson's disease;

provide financial counseling, such as evaluating insurance plans and investments, budgeting, reconciling debt;

assist with drafting living wills, wills, powers of attorney, etc.; filling out Medicare, Social Security, and health care claims forms; analyzing retirement pension/benefits.

Cross-Reference: Chapter 23, Senior Fairs; Chapter 49, Programs and Activities for the Stages of Life; Chapter 51, Programs and Activities for Staying Connected

51 Programs and Activities for Staying Connected

One regrettable trait of Americans approaching the twenty-first century is that we have become increasingly isolated, both physically and emotionally, from our fellow humans . . . even within our own families. For the older citizen, this distancing has become profound. Wellness programs can become the conduit for reestablishing many of these connections.

The impact of isolation and loss on depression in aging audiences cannot be overemphasized. Grown children may live many miles away and have their own interests. Older friends and loved ones may be dead or incapacitated. New technologies are bewildering, even frightening. Often, health problems are at least an indirect result of these emotional stresses.

Goals

To provide a safe environment for people seeking the companionship of others their age or those with similar interests

To provide the necessary skills to reach out to others

To rekindle old passions and establish new interests

Target audience

All types, middle-age and older

Process

- Make sure the facility is fully accessible.
- Offer programs and classes for lifelong learning:

  Computer classes: Help people rekindle old relationships through writing letters more easily; connects people to the wonders of the Internet (not the least of which is the ability to "talk" to people around the world with similar interests); provides them the new tools for managing personal affairs, or supplementing their income

  Pet care and training: The value of pets in bringing people out of themselves is well established. A trained, well-cared for pet gives the owner greater pleasure and is easier for an aging owner to keep for as long as possible.

Gardening tips for flowers and vegetables: Caring for and nurturing plants to maturity establishes a valuable connection to the outside world through nature.

Creative writing programs: Translating long-forgotten memories and repressed emotions onto paper helps bring people out of themselves and into the present. Journaling can be done at home, but group programs encourage sharing of feelings and interests.

Genealogy classes: Help participants connect to past generations.

- Sponsor social events:

  card games: bridge, poker, cribbage, gin rummy, etc.

  ballroom dances

  storytelling night: a "shared reminiscing" night, where people take turns sharing memories on various topics selected by them or a facilitator or take turns telling the biggest lie (give a prize at the end of the evening for the "biggest whopper")

  movie nights: old movies shown on a VCR

- Help your audience reach out to others less fortunate:

  support local charities by forwarding the proceeds from sponsored bake sales with products made by participants, sponsored arts and crafts fairs with items made by participants, sales of quilts created at ongoing quilting parties;

  open a thrift shop: participants donate items for selling, but also get together to help renovate donated items (for instance, tearing cloth scraps and making them into rugs and other items, replacing lost stones and polishing old costume jewelry, putting puzzles together to make sure all the pieces are present, cleaning old collector bottles, etc.), volunteer in running the shop, and donate proceeds;

  sponsor trips to children's hospitals, orphanages, and day-care centers so participants can tell stories to the children;

  set up visiting programs where participants can read books or the newspaper to shut-ins and the visually impaired.

Cross-Reference: Chapter 23, Senior Fairs; Chapter 49, Programs and Activities for the Stages of Life; Chapter 50, Programs and Activities for Encouraging Independence and Safety

Resources

Catalogues

Childbirth Graphics, a division of WRS Group, Inc., PO Box 21207, Waco, TX 76702-1207, Ph: 800-299-3366, ext. 287 (source for: pregnancy pillow, folding displays, smoking and pregnancy models, posters, breast self-exam models)

Great Performance, 14964 NW Greenbrier Parkway, Beaverton, OR 97006, Ph: 800-433-3803 (source for: posters)

Health Edco, a division of WRS Group, Inc., PO Box 21207, Waco, TX 76702-1207, Ph: 800-299-3366, ext. 295 (source for: folding displays, smoking and pregnancy models, cancerous/emphysemic lung models, anatomical models, mouth models on effects of oral tobacco, breast self-exam models, pregnancy pillows, plastic food models)

Johnson and Johnson Health Management, Inc., 410 George Street, New Brunswick, NJ 08901, Ph: 800-443-3682 (source for: general and focused health-risk appraisals)

Loose Change Product, Financial Literacy Center, 350 East Michigan Ave., Suite 301, Kalamazoo, MI 49007, Ph: 888-679-3300, ext. 1285 (source for: financial health material)

Nasco, 901 Janesville Ave., Fort Atkinson, WI 53538-0901, Ph: 414-563-2446 (source for: pregnancy pillows, infant simulator dolls, folding displays, drug identification displays, smoking and pregnancy models, cancerous/emphysemic lung models, mouth models on effects of oral tobacco, plastic food models, anatomical models)

Visual Horizons, 180 Metro Park, Rochester, New York 14623-2666, Ph: 716-424-5300 (source for: photographic and cartoon 35mm slides and overhead transparencies to incorporate in presentations)

Whole Person Associates, 210 West Michigan, Duluth, MN 55802-1908, Ph: 800-247-6789 (source for: structured exercise books with icebreaker activities)

Other References

"Health Hotlines" (NIH Publication 96-2780), National Library of Medicine/SIS, 8600 Rockville Pike, Bethesda, MD 20894, Ph: 301-496-3147

Compilation of organizations with toll-free telephone numbers. This database contains descriptions of more than 17,000 biomedical information resources, including organizations, databases, research resources, etc. Some of the subject areas included in "Health Hotlines" are AIDS, cancer, maternal and child health, aging, substance abuse, disabilities, and mental health. "Health Hotlines" also lists a variety of groups disseminating information on a number of specific diseases and disorders. Organizations fall into many categories, including federal, state, and local government agencies; information and referral centers; professional societies; support groups; and voluntary associations.

"Healthy People 2000," ODHP Communication Support Center, PO Box 37366, Washington, DC 20013-7366

Reference for government health goals for America, including statistics on various ethnic groups, ages, and gender health risks.

International Institute for Health Promotion, (Attention Wolf Kirsten), National Center for Health Fitness, American University, 4400 Massachusetts Avenue NW, Washington DC 20016-8037, Internet site: www.healthy.american.edu/iihpconsort.html, Ph: 202-885-6275

American University has committed considerable time, resources, and financial support to the formation of the Institute, resulting in the establishment of a worldwide network in the field of health promotion. This organization may be helpful in developing strategies for bringing health promotion services to corporate or government sites overseas.

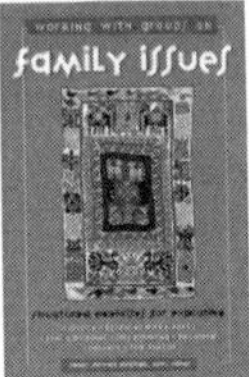

WORKING WITH GROUPS ON FAMILY ISSUES

Sandy Stewart Christian, MSW, LICSW, Editor

These 24 structured exercises combine the knowledge of marriage and family experts with practical techniques to help you move individuals, couples, and families toward positive change. Topics include divorce, single parenting, stepfamilies, gay and lesbian relationships, working partners, and more.

- ❑ **Working with Groups on Family Issues / $24.95**
- ❑ **Worksheet Masters / $9.95**

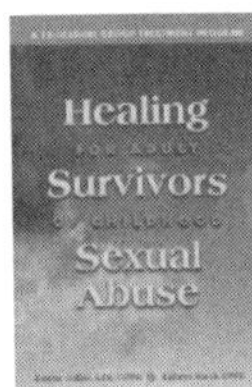

HEALING FOR ADULT SURVIVORS OF CHILDHOOD SEXUAL ABUSE

Bonnie Collins, EdM, CSW-R, and Kathryn Marsh, CSW-R

As many as 20 percent of girls are sexually abused. In this manual, you will find a complete 12-session program for treating clients whose problems stem from the sexual abuse they experienced as children.

- ❑ **Healing for Adult Survivors of Childhood Sexual Abuse / $24.95**
- ❑ **Worksheet Masters / $9.95**

WORKING WITH GROUPS IN THE WORKPLACE

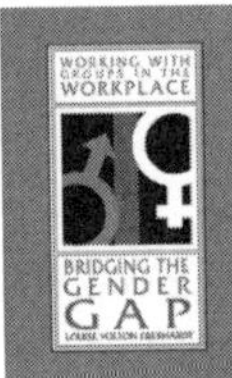

BRIDGING THE GENDER GAP

Louise Yolton Eberhardt

Bridging the Gender Gap contains a wealth of exercises for trainers to use in gender role awareness groups, diversity training, couples workshops, college classes, and youth seminars.

- ❑ **Bridging the Gender Gap / $24.95**
- ❑ **Worksheet Masters / $9.95**

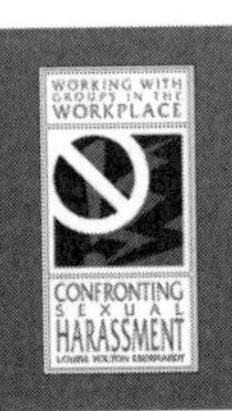

CONFRONTING SEXUAL HARASSMENT

Louise Yolton Eberhardt

Confronting Sexual Harassment presents exercises that trainers can safely use with groups to constructively explore the issues of sexual harassment, look at the underlying causes, understand the law, motivate men to become allies, and empower women to speak up.

- ❑ **Confronting Sexual Harassment / $24.95**
- ❑ **Worksheet Masters / $9.95**

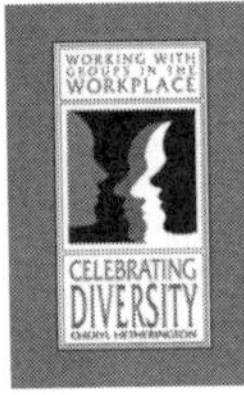

CELEBRATING DIVERSITY

Cheryl Hetherington

Celebrating Diversity helps people confront and question the beliefs, prejudices, and fears that can separate them from others. Carefully written exercises help trainers present these sensitive issues in the workplace as well as in educational settings.

- ❑ **Celebrating Diversity / $24.95**
- ❑ **Worksheet Masters / $9.95**

Call 1-800-247-6789 to receive a catalog or to place an order for any Whole Person Associates product.

MIND-BODY MAGIC

Martha Belknap, MA

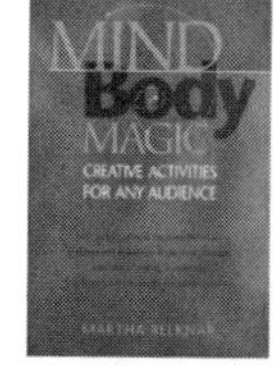

Make any presentation more powerful with one of these 40 feel-good activities. Handy tips with each activity show you how to use it in your presentation, plus ideas for enhancing or extending the activity, and suggestions for adapting it for your teaching goals and audience. Use *Mind-Body Magic* to present any topic with pizzazz!

❑ **Mind-Body Magic / $21.95**
❑ **Worksheet Masters / $9.95**

INSTANT ICEBREAKERS

50 Powerful Catalysts for Group Interaction and High-Impact Learning

Sandy Stewart Christian, MSW, and
Nancy Loving Tubesing, EdD, Editors

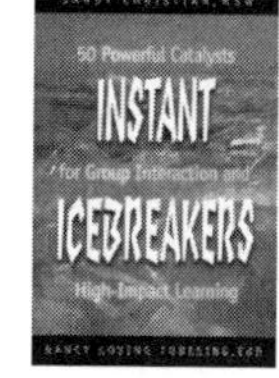

Introduce the subject at hand and introduce participants to each other with these proven strategies that apply to all kinds of audiences and appeal to many learning styles. Step-by-step instructions make any presentation a breeze.

❑ **Instant Icebreakers / $24.95**
❑ **Worksheet Masters / $9.95**

PLAYING ALONG

37 Group Learning Activities Borrowed from Improvisational Theater

Izzy Gesell, MS

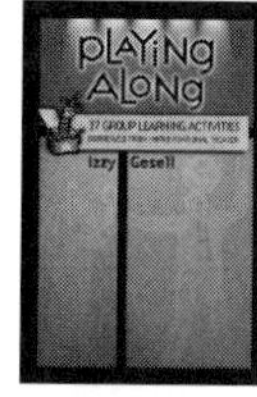

Set the stage for learning and growth with these innovative, playful activities borrowed from a classic art form: improvisational theater. Whatever your topic, these brief (5-10 minute) exercises activate the all-important learning skills of listening, accepting, affirming, imagining, and trusting—and pave the way for personal growth or organizational change.

❑ **Playing Along / $21.95**

CREATING A CLIMATE FOR POWER LEARNING

37 Mind-Stretching Activities

Carolyn Chambers Clark, EdD, ARNP

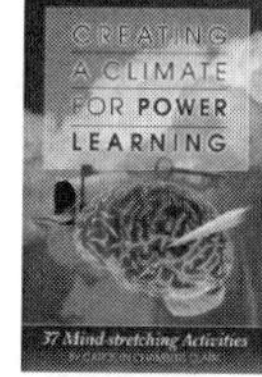

Creative warm-up processes that prepare leaders and participants for a satisfying learning experience. These activities will enhance your presentation skills, leadership style, and teaching effectiveness no matter what your audience or setting.

❑ **Creating a Climate for Power Learning / $21.95**

PLAYFUL ACTIVITIES FOR POWERFUL PRESENTATIONS

Bruce Williamson

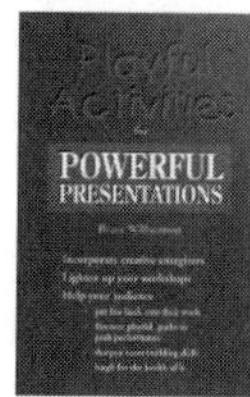

Spice up presentations with healthy laughter. The 40 creative energizers in this book will enhance learning, stimulate communication, promote teamwork, and reduce resistance to group interaction.

❑ **Playful Activities for Powerful Presentations / $24.95**

Call 1-800-247-6789 to receive a catalog or to place an order for any Whole Person Associates product.

ADDITIONAL GROUP PROCESS RESOURCES

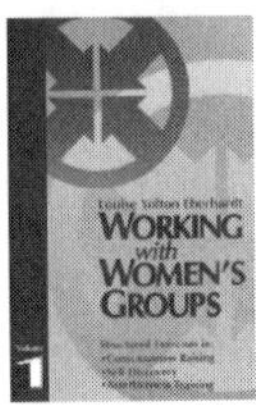

WORKING WITH WOMEN'S GROUPS VOLUMES 1 & 2

Louise Yolton Eberhardt

When leading a women's group, don't just rely on personal experience and intuition—equip yourself with these volumes of proven exercises. Louise Yolton Eberhardt has distilled more than a quarter century of experience into nearly a hundred processes addressing the issues that are most important to women today.

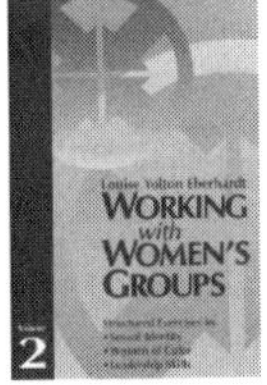

The two volumes of *Working with Women's Groups* have been completely revised and updated. *Volume 1* explores consciousness raising, self-discovery, and assertiveness training. *Volume 2* looks at sexuality issues, women of color, and leadership skills training.

- ❑ **Working with Women's Groups, Vols. 1 & 2 / $24.95 each**
- ❑ **Worksheet Masters, Vols. 1 & 2 / $9.95 each**

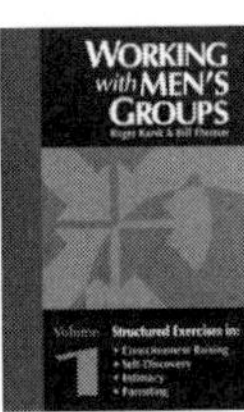

WORKING WITH MEN'S GROUPS

Roger Karsk and Bill Thomas

Working with Men's Groups has been updated to reflect the reality of men's lives in the 1990s. Each exercise follows a structured pattern to help trainers develop either onetime workshops or ongoing groups that explore men's issues in four key areas: self-discovery, consciousness raising, intimacy, and parenting.

- ❑ **Working with Men's Groups / $24.95**
- ❑ **Worksheet Masters / $9.95**

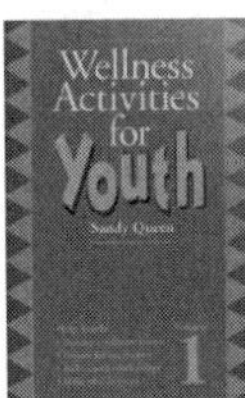

WELLNESS ACTIVITIES FOR YOUTH VOLUMES 1 & 2

Sandy Queen

Each volume of *Wellness Activities for Youth* provides 36 complete classroom activities that help leaders teach children and teenagers about wellness with a whole person approach and an emphasis on FUN. The concepts include: values, stress and coping, self-esteem, personal well-being, and social wellness.

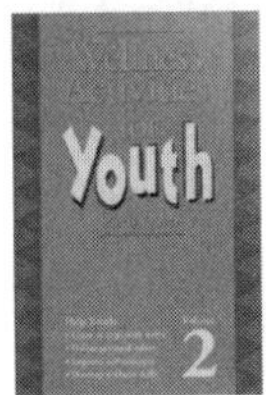

Curriculum developer Sandy Queen designed these whole-person "no-put-down" activities for kids from middle school to high school age, but many can be adapted for families or even for the corporate setting.

- ❑ **Wellness Activities for Youth, Vols. 1 & 2 / $21.95 each**
- ❑ **Worksheet Masters, Vols. 1 & 2 / $9.95 each**

Call 1-800-247-6789 to receive a catalog or to place an order for any Whole Person Associates product.

TOPICAL GROUP RESOURCES

WORKING WITH GROUPS ON SPIRITUAL THEMES

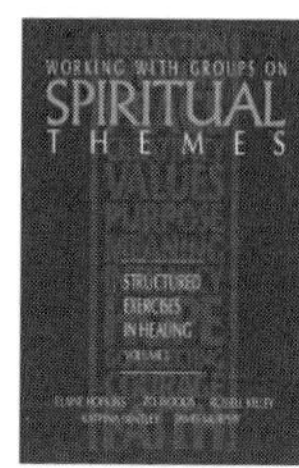

Elaine Hopkins, Zo Woods, Russell Kelley, Katrina Bentley, and James Murphy

True wellness must address the spirit. Many groups that originally form around issues such as physical or mental health, stress management, or relationships eventually recognize the importance of spiritual issues. The material contained in this manual helps health professionals initiate discussion on spiritual needs in a logical, organized fashion that induces a high level of comfort for group members and leaders.

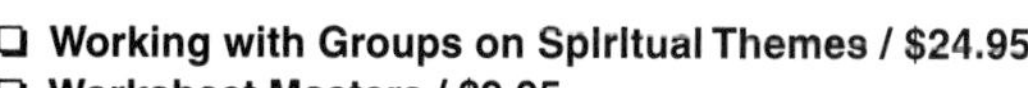

❑ **Working with Groups on Spiritual Themes / $24.95**
❑ **Worksheet Masters / $9.95**

WORKING WITH GROUPS TO OVERCOME PANIC, ANXIETY, & PHOBIAS

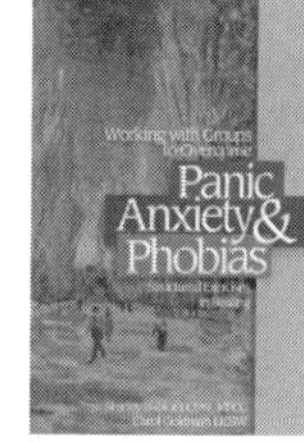

Shirley Babior, LCSW, MFCC, and Carol Goldman, LICSW

Written especially for therapists, this manual presents well-researched, state-of-the-art treatment strategies for a variety of anxiety disorders. It includes treatment goals, basic anxiety-recovery exercises, and recovery enhancers that encourage lifestyle changes. Sessions in this manual are related directly to the chapters in *Overcoming Panic, Anxiety, & Phobias.*

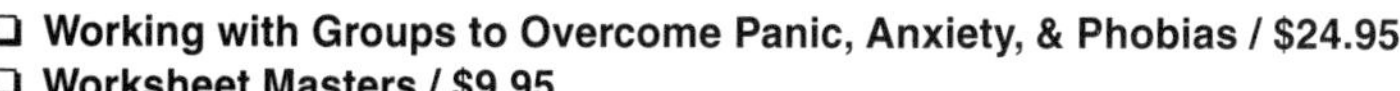

❑ **Working with Groups to Overcome Panic, Anxiety, & Phobias / $24.95**
❑ **Worksheet Masters / $9.95**

WORKING WITH GROUPS TO EXPLORE FOOD & BODY CONNECTIONS

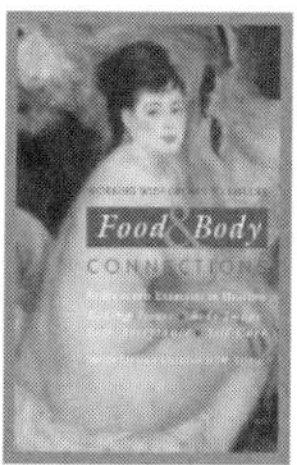

Sandy Stewart Christian, MSW, Editor

This collection of 36 group processes gathered from experts around the country tackles complex and painful issues nearly everyone is concerned about—dieting, weight, healthy eating, fitness, body image, and self-esteem—using a whole person approach that advocates health and fitness for people of all sizes.

❑ **Working with Groups to Explore Food & Body Connections / $24.95**
❑ **Worksheet Masters / $9.95**

CREATIVE PLANNING FOR THE SECOND HALF OF LIFE

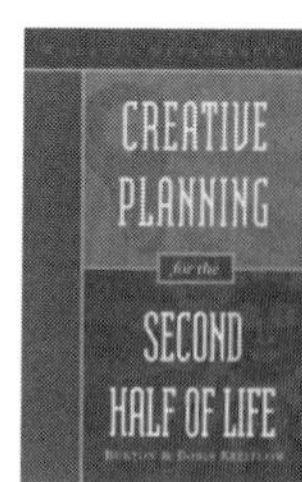

Burton Kreitlow, PhD, and Doris Kreitlow, MS

This is the first book to help group leaders design a presentation or workshop that addresses the whole-person needs of people ages 50 and up. These 29 structured exercises explore ways of planning for retirement by finding intriguing ways to make a useful life for yourself—not simply setting aside money for the day you quit working.

❑ **Creative Planning for the Second Half of Life / $24.95**
❑ **Worksheet Masters / $9.95**